Case Studies in
Occupational
Epidemiology

Case Studies
in Occupational
Epidemiology

Edited by

KYLE STEENLAND

New York   Oxford
OXFORD UNIVERSITY PRESS
1993

Oxford University Press

Oxford   New York   Toronto
Delhi   Bombay   Calcutta   Madras   Karachi
Kuala Lumpur   Singapore   Hong Kong   Tokyo
Nairobi   Dar es Salaam   Cape Town
Melbourne   Auckland   Madrid

and associated companies in
Berlin   Ibadan

Library of Congress Catalog-in-Publication Data
Case studies in occupational epidemiology / edited by Kyle Steenland.
p. cm.   Includes bibliographical references and index.
ISBN 0-19-506831-9
1. Occupational diseases—Epidemiology—Case studies.
2. Occupational diseases—Epidemiology—Examinations, questions, etc.
I. Steenland, Kyle, 1946–   .
[DNLM: 1. Epidemiologic Methods—problems.
2. Occupational Diseases—epidemiology—problems.
WA 18 C337]
RC964.C285   1993
614.4'0722—dc20   DNLM/DLC
for Library of Congress   92-6175

1 2 3 4 5 6 7 8 9

Printed in the United States of America
on acid-free paper

Preface

The purpose of this book is to provide material for teaching epidemiology. Thirteen case studies are arranged in four parts (cohort studies, case-control and proportionate mortality studies, cross-sectional studies, and surveillance and screening studies). Each part begins with a description of the general study design. The case studies are based on actual epidemiologic studies and have been written by the respective principal investigators. It is hoped that they preserve the flavor of the practical problems confronted by the working epidemiologist.

A broad range of etiologic studies is considered, and all major study designs are well represented. In addition, the chapters on surveillance give the reader practical examples of how public health practitioners can use surveillance data to develop effective interventions. The case study on screening illustrates the issues involved in screening a population at high risk of bladder cancer due to occupational exposure.

The book deals with a wide variety of disease outcomes, including spontaneous abortion, carpal tunnel syndrome, kidney dysfunction, cytogenetic changes, ischemic heart disease, dermatitis, chronic renal disease, and several types of cancer. The exposures of interest are equally diverse, including VDT use, repetitive hand-wrist motion, heavy metals, carbon monoxide, diesel exhaust, lead, vinyl chloride, pesticides, solvents, silica, and acid mists. These outcomes and exposures represent many of the current topics of interest in occupational health.

While the case studies are occupational in nature, the principles involved are the same as for any type of epidemiologic study. Thus, the book can be used in general courses on epidemiology as well as in higher-level courses on occupational epidemiology.

Each case study, arranged in the same format, attempts to take the reader through the same steps that the investigator took when conducting the actual study. The student is asked to solve the same problems that the investigator solved in the course of the study. Each case study includes questions regarding study design, identification and measurement of exposure, problems of data collection, analytical issues, and issues of interpretation. Answers are provided at the end of each chapter. Many of the cases also include analytical exercises suitable for classroom use.

The book is designed so that most calculations can be done with a pocket calculator. Measures and statistics required for answering analytical questions in the text are presented in the Appendix. Optional questions based on multivariate analyses using either linear or logistic regression (requiring a computer) are also offered in several of the case studies.

Data sets are attached to five of the case studies. For three others the data sets were too large to include in the text. However, course instructors using this text may obtain all eight data sets as ASCI files on diskette from the editor.

This book is a collaborative effort. Seven of the case studies have been written by other investigators, albeit with some editing by myself. I bear sole responsibility for six of the studies, as well as for the introductions and the Appendix. Alberto Salvan and Deanna Wild kindly helped check some of the calculations.

Cincinnati, Ohio   K. S.
May 1992

Contents

Contributors

MICHAEL O'MALLEY, MD, MPH
California Environmental Protection Agency
Department of Pesticide Regulation
Sacramento, California

ANA OSORIO, MD, MPH
California Department of Health Services
Berkeley, California

TERESA SCHNORR, PhD
National Institute for Occupational Safety and Health
Cincinnati, Ohio

KYLE STEENLAND, PhD
National Institute for Occupational Safety and Health
Cincinnati, Ohio

FRANK STERN, MS
National Institute for Occupational Safety and Health
Cincinnati, Ohio

MICHAEL THUN, MD, MS
American Cancer Society
Atlanta, Georgia

ELIZABETH WARD, PhD
National Institute for Occupational Safety and Health
Cincinnati, Ohio

Case Studies in
Occupational
Epidemiology

Part I | Cohort Studies

In a cohort study the investigator defines a cohort of nondiseased, exposed individuals and a cohort of nondiseased, nonexposed individuals (the comparison or referent population) and follows them over time to determine disease incidence. Cohort studies can be either prospective or retrospective. In a prospective study the subjects are identified in the present and followed into the future. For example, a sample of the population of Framingham, Massachusetts, free of heart disease and aged 30–59, was enrolled in 1950–1952 in a now famous prospective study (Dawber et al., 1951). A variety of risk factors for heart disease were measured at that time (enabling investigators to divide the population by "exposure" status, such as high blood pressure versus low blood pressure). The population has since been followed to determine the incidence of heart disease.

Retrospective cohort studies identify exposed and nonexposed populations at some point in the past and then determine who among them has developed disease. For example, to determine the association between carbon monoxide and heart disease, workers exposed to carbon monoxide while working in tollbooths outside the entrances to tunnels of Manhattan before 1965 were identified by government investigators in the mid-1980s (Stern et al., 1988). Their heart disease mortality through 1984 was subsequently determined and then compared to the general population of a similar age, race, and sex distribution. Retrospective cohort studies are often advantageous because the investigator does not need to wait many years for an appreciable number of individuals to get the disease of interest. On the other hand, in retrospective cohort studies investigators are often unable to obtain precise information on level of exposure or other risk factors (e.g., blood pressure or smoking) since the exposure occurred in the past, and since the cohort may now be dispersed and difficult to contact.

Cohort studies are most useful in the study of rare exposures and common diseases. Rare exposures can be studied by choosing the specific group that has been exposed, even if the exposure is uncommon in the general population. For example, exposure to vinyl chloride gas is uncommon in the general population, but one could study one or several manufacturing plants where vinyl chloride is produced to obtain a fairly large population. Rare diseases are a problem in cohort studies, because even if a large cohort is assembled only a few cases may occur, limiting the ability of the investigator to detect a difference between exposed and nonexposed groups. Suppose, for example, that one wanted to study end-stage renal disease among workers exposed to solvents. A cohort of solvent-exposed workers might have to number in the hundreds of thousands for many cases of end-stage renal disease (male incidence about 10/100,000) to be observed.

Cohort studies also have the advantage that more than one disease can be studied, so that the possible association of the exposure of interest with a given disease can be evaluated for a multitude of diseases simultaneously. Even though a particular exposure–disease association has been hypothesized a priori, a posteriori data analysis may uncover unexpected exposure–disease associations.

Cohort studies may address either the proportion of the study population exposed over time (cumulative incidence) or the rate of disease among the study population (incidence rate, or incidence density rate). The former measure is based on "count" data while the latter measure uses person-time data. Consider the data for the five hypothetical individuals below:

```
     0        1        2        3        4        5 years
1 _____ * disease
2 _____
3 _____ * disease
4 _____
5 _____
```

Cumulative incidence is defined as follows:

$$\text{C.I.} = \frac{\text{Number of new cases of disease during a defined period}}{\text{Total number of people at risk of disease}}$$

The incidence rate is defined as follows:

$$\frac{\text{Number of new cases of disease during a defined period}}{\text{Person-time at risk}}$$

In this example, the cumulative incidence is 2/5, or 0.40, while the incidence rate is 2 cases/19 person-years at risk, or 0.11. With incidence rates individuals can enter the study at any time, can contribute unequal numbers of person-years, and can also be lost to follow-up before the study end. Cumulative incidence, on the other hand, is often calculated in situations where everyone is followed for the same length of time with minimal or no loss to follow-up. Cumulative incidence is most appropriate for studies with short follow-up periods. When considering the disease incidence in an exposed and versus a nonexposed population, relative risks may be calculated from cumulative incidence data while rate ratios may be calculated from incidence rates.

Three cohort studies are described in Part I. The first is a retrospective cumulative incidence study of spontaneous abortion among women working with video display terminals (VDTs). The follow-up period in this study is only a few years. The second is a retrospective cohort mortality study of workers exposed to carbon monoxide, focusing on heart disease as the outcome of interest. The third is a retrospective cohort incidence study of larynx cancer among men exposed to sulfuric acid. Both the second and the third studies involve long follow-up periods and are based on person-time data.

References

Dawber T, Meadors F, Moore F. Epidemiologic approaches to heart disease: the Framingham Study. Am J Public Heath 41: 279–286, 1951.

Stern F, Halperin W, Hornung R. Heart disease mortality among bridge and tunnel officers exposed to carbon monoxide. Am J Epidemiol, 128, 6: 1276–1288, 1988.

Chapter 1 Video Display Terminals and Adverse Pregnancy Outcomes

TERESA SCHNORR

Video display terminals (VDTs) were first associated with adverse reproductive outcomes in 1980, when a cluster of birth defects was observed among women using VDTs at the Toronto *Star* newspaper. This report was followed by a number of other adverse pregnancy outcome clusters, primarily spontaneous abortion, but including other adverse outcomes such as stillbirths, low birthweight, and preterm birth (Berquist, 1984).

Three different hypotheses were proposed as possible explanations for the clusters: (1) physical stress (defined as prolonged sitting), (2) psychological stress due to the demands of the work environment, and (3) electromagnetic energy emissions (Tell, 1990). As of 1984, no epidemiologic studies of VDT and pregnancy outcome study were underway in the United States, and the literature contained little information on the potential hazards of VDTs. While physical stress, defined as heavy lifting, had been associated with an increased risk of preterm birth (Mamelle et al., 1984), the association with work posture (sitting versus standing) had not been studied. There was little information about the potential effect of workplace psychological stress on reproductive function, although two studies had shown an association between a measure of occupational mental stress and premature birth (Mamelle et al., 1984; Naeye and Peters, 1982). No animal or human studies had been conducted of the potential reproductive hazards of electromagnetic fields produced by VDTs. These electromagnetic fields were of two types, ELF (extra-low frequency) and VLF (very low frequency). These two frequencies are in the lower end of the electromagnetic spectrum, below radio waves or microwaves. ELF fields are also produced by common 60 Hz wiring in houses and appliances. Studies of the reproductive effects in animals exposed to ELF and VLF were just beginning.

Because of the large number of women using VDTs in the workplace and the public concern, the National Institute for Occupational Safety and Health

(NIOSH) decided to conduct a study to determine if VDTs posed a risk for pregnant women. The focus was to be on spontaneous abortions, but researchers wanted to investigate other possible adverse outcomes as well (low birthweight, birth defects, stillbirth, and preterm birth).

QUESTION 1. What would be the most appropriate design for a study of spontaneous abortion and other outcomes among VDT users: case-control, prospective cohort, or retrospective cohort? How would you determine the outcome(s) for each type of study?

QUESTION 2. What would be your principal definition of exposure for a study of spontaneous abortions among VDT users? How would your study design take into account all the hypothesized exposures of interest (electromagnetic fields, physical and psychological stress)?

QUESTION 3. How would you calculate the estimated number of women needed in the exposed and nonexposed populations (assume a 1-to-1 ratio) for the proposed study design? Sketch out an approach to the answer; you do not need to do actual calculations.

QUESTION 4. What are the important confounders to consider in such a study?

Materials and Methods

The investigators decided to conduct a cohort study in a population of telephone operators. Reproductive histories were to be obtained via telephone interview. Medical confirmation of reported spontaneous abortions would be sought.

One type of operator, the directory assistance operator, used a VDT for the entire work day. The comparison group was made up of general operators who did not use VDTs. Both groups shared the same degree of physical and psychological stress.

Directory assistance operators used the VDT to locate telephone directory information and provide it to customers who called in. A computer automatically routed incoming calls to the next available operator, so the time between calls was brief. Operators usually had less than a second between calls. Operators were monitored by the computer, which recorded their number and length of calls. They were also monitored by their supervisors.

The general operator, the operator reached by dialing "0," had duties similar to those of the directory assistance operator. General operators assisted customers in placing long-distance calls, among other duties. General operators did not use a VDT; they used a light-emitting diode (LED) or neon glow tube (NIXIE tube) screen. Like the directory assistance operators, the general operators were monitored by a computer and by their supervisors, and calls were automatically routed to the next available operator so that the time between calls was usually less than a second.

Both jobs required the same education and skills, and salaries were similar. Both operator groups had duties that required that they sit for seven hours a day in front of their respective equipment. Both groups also had jobs that included customer contact and both machine and human monitoring. While there may have been some differences in work practices between the two groups, the primary difference was the presence or absence of the VDT.

Two companies with both exposed and nonexposed operators were tentatively identified for the study. A study period was defined as 1/1/83–7/1/86.

There were 5,544 operators (exposed and nonexposed) employed between these dates at the two companies. To maximize the number of pregnancies, women were required to have been between 18 and 33 years of age during the study period. To be eligible for the study, a woman had to have been employed and married at some point during this period. Furthermore, the operator had to have been pregnant and employed for at least one day during the first 28 weeks of gestation, and the pregnancy had to terminate between January 1, 1983, and December 1, 1986 (the follow-up period). The date of the last menstrual period, obtained during interview, was considered the beginning date of each pregnancy.

Addresses and telephone numbers of potential study participants were obtained from company records. Addresses were checked against post office and IRS records to obtain updated addresses. A letter describing the study and requesting participation was sent to each potential participant. This letter was followed up by a phone call in which it was determined whether the woman had been married during the study period, and if she had been pregnant while employed at the company. If so, a 25-minute home telephone interview was conducted, in which a reproductive history during the study period was obtained.

Unfortunately, approximately 50% of the cohort had outdated telephone numbers. Locating current phone numbers was hampered by two factors: (1) women tended to list their phone numbers under their husbands' names, and (2) a benefit of working for the phone company was receiving an unlisted phone number at no extra charge. Investigators found 40% of the missing phone numbers through directory assistance, often using information on the husband's first name which was received in the IRS verification process.

QUESTION 5. How would you go about obtaining phone numbers for the remaining 30% of the cohort.

QUESTION 6. How would you define a spontaneous abortion? What would you do about induced abortions? Ectopic pregnancies? Twins?

Results

The full results of this study can be found in Schnorr et al. (1991).

After extensive tracing efforts, 19.3% of the potential participants still could not be contacted. Another 3.3% refused to participate.

Based on the interview data, investigators found 366 pregnancies among director assistance (DA) operators and 516 pregnancies to general operators during the follow-up period (1/1/83–1/1/86). The number of spontaneous abortions (SABs) by month of gestation and VDT exposure status are given in Table 1.1.

QUESTION 7. Calculate the crude SAB rate and relative risk for VDT-exposed pregnancies. Also calculate the SAB rate by month of gestation for each group. What are your findings from this initial review?

Table 1.2 gives the results for the study pregnancies stratified by history of SAB and smoking status at time of pregnancy, the two best-known risk factors.

QUESTION 8. Calculate a Mantel-Haenszel relative risk for SAB for the exposed versus the nonexposed from Table 1.2, and its confidence interval. Does it appear that prior SAB and smoking act as confounders?

A simple analysis of exposed versus nonexposed might obscure a trend of increasing risk with increasing exposure. Table 1.3 gives the data by categories of hours of VDT use during the first 28 weeks of pregnancy (although exposed women worked generally full-time with VDTs, hours varied depending on vacations, sick leave, whether a woman was hired when already pregnant, etc.). An adjustment was made to account for the fact that pregnancies ending in SAB

TABLE 1.1 Spontaneous Abortions by Exposure Status and Gestational Month

Month of Gestation	Unexposed Pregnancies No. of SABs	Exposed Pregnancies No. of SABs
1	10	1
2	38	30
3	15	12
4	7	5
5	2	4
6	4	1
7	2	1
Unknown	4	0
Total SABs	82	54
Total Pregnancies	516	366

TABLE 1.2 Spontaneous Abortions Stratified by Risk Factors

	Unexposed Pregnancy		Exposed Pregnancy	
	SAB	No SAB	SAB	No SAB
Prior SAB, smoker	3	13	3	13
Prior SAB, nonsmoker	11	29	7	28
No prior SAB, smoker	20	78	14	62
No prior SAB, nonsmoker	48	311	30	209

would have fewer VDT hours while pregnant than pregnancies not ending in SAB (for details see Schnorr et al., 1991).

QUESTION 9. Calculate the relative risks for SAB for 1–25 hours and for 25+ hours. Is there an apparent trend with increasing hours of VDT use? Calculate the Mantel chi-square test for trend, using as category scores 0 hours, 12.5 hours, and 30 hours. What is the chi-square and what is its p-value?

Investigators then conducted a logistic regression analysis of the data, evaluating each of the potential covariates for confounding and interaction with VDT use. Important predictors of the final model included cigarette smoking (amount per day and yes/no), prior spontaneous abortion (0/1), and presence of a thyroid disorder prior to pregnancy (0/1). Also included were the average number of hours per week (0 for the nonexposed).

QUESTION 10 (optional). Course instructors may obtain the study data (VDT.DAT) on a diskette from the editor. There are 882 observations and seven variables on the file. The variables (in order) are average VDT hours in first trimester, the number of cigarettes per day, prior SAB, SAB, smoking status (yes/no), prior thyroid condition, and VDT exposure in first trimester (yes/no). All dichotomous variables are coded 1 for yes, 0 for no. Note that a number of observations have missing values for hours per week of VDT exposure.

TABLE 1.3 Spontaneous Abortion and Frequency of VDT Use

VDT Use in First 28 Weeks (hr/wk)	SAB	No SAB	Total
None (general operators)	78	416	494
1–25	22	97	119
25+	26	153	179

As an optional exercise, use logistic regression with the data on VDT.DAT to estimate the odds ratio of SAB for exposed versus nonexposed controlling for the other predictors of SAB. Does the adjusted odds ratio differ substantially from the "cruder" Mantel-Haenszel relative risk calculated above? Test whether there are any interactions between exposure and other predictor variables. Test for an increasing trend of SAB risk with increased VDT exposure (hours per week), and with increased cigarette smoking. Is there a significant trend for either variable?

QUESTION 11. The analyses performed in this study assume that all outcomes are independent events. However, 125 (17%) of the women had more than one study pregnancy. What could be done to determine if these non-independent events affected the findings?

QUESTION 12. Induced abortions were excluded from the analysis. What is the potential bias that could result if there is a difference in the rate or the timing of induced abortion between the two groups? What can be done to determine if this is a potential problem?

Information on the outcomes of pregnancy was reported by the women themselves. Thus, there is a possibility of differences in recall between the groups. According to the interviews, virtually all reported SABs were also reported by the study participant to their physician (only ten were not). Investigators were given permission by study participants to obtain medical records on only a very small number of SABs, so the interview data could not be verified directly. However, a confidential portion of the birth certificate contains information on the number of prior terminations (including SABs) and live births for the mother (Mausner and Bahn, 1974). This confidential section of the certificate is not available to the public, but NIOSH researchers were able to obtain it for research purposes.

QUESTION 13. How could this information be used to determine if women were reporting SABs accurately, and whether there were any reporting differences between exposed and nonexposed groups?

Two models of VDT were used by the directory assistance operators during the study period: an International Business Machines (IBM) model and a Computer Consoles, Inc. (CCI) model. NIOSH researchers visited eight of the 50 offices where the directory assistance operators worked and measured the electromagnetic fields at six randomly selected VDTs at each site for a total of 48 VDTs (24 IBM and 24 CCI). They also measured fields at 24 of the light-emitting diode (LED) units and 24 of the neon glow tube units. Several measurements were made. First, researchers measured the ELF and VLF electric (E−) and magnetic (H−) fields at 30 cm from each of the six surfaces of the VDT and non-VDT units. Second, these same measurements were conducted at the operator's normal position in front of the unit (approximately 80–100 cm). Third, researchers measured the current that was induced to flow through the operator when she was in contact with the unit. Geometric means and geometric standard deviations for a sample of these measurements are given in Table 1.4, which shows that, at 30 cm, the VDTs had significantly higher levels of electromagnetic fields than did the non-VDT units. Women using the non-VDT units had virtually no VLF electromagnetic field exposure. The women using the non-VDT units had some exposure to ELF fields. The CCI model of VDT emitted higher levels than did the IBM.

At the operator's normal position there was less difference in exposure between VDT and non-VDT units. The operator generally sits farther than 30 cm from the VDT, and exposure drops sharply at increasing distance. For ELF magnetic fields, there was no significant difference in exposure levels between general and directory assistance operators when measurements were recorded at the operators' normal working position. Measurements were then conducted of the spatial variation of the fields (not shown in this study) (Tell, 1990), and these showed that the ELF exposure levels of the general operators did not

TABLE 1.4 Geometric Mean (GM) and Geometric Standard Deviation (GSD) of Electromagnetic Energy Measurements

	Very Low Frequency (VLF), GM (GSD)*		Extremely Low Frequency (ELF), GM (GSD)	
	E-Field (V/m)	H-Field (mA/m)	E-Field (V/m)	H-Field (mA/m)
Unit Type				
Frontal Emissions (30 cm)				
VDT				
CCI	4.2 (1.54)[†]	98.9 (2.61)[†]	1.9 (1.63)[†]	313.6 (1.22)[†]
IBM	3.3 (2.07)	22.1 (4.68)	1.8 (1.93)	236.1 (2.14)
Non-VDT				
LED	0.1 (1.16)	1.6 (1.01)	0.4 (1.10)	72.3 (1.68)
NGT	0.1 (2.05)	1.4 (1.04)	0.5 (1.40)	30.3 (1.72)
Abdominal Exposure (80–100 cm)				
VDT				
CCI	0.5 (1.68)[†]	17.4 (1.74)[†]	0.8 (3.61)[†]	62.3 (1.59)
IBM	0.1 (1.71)	4.0 (1.85)	0.4 (1.70)	57.7 (2.12)
Non-VDT				
LED	0.1 (1.35)	2.0 (1.15)	0.4 (1.18)	62.4 (2.79)
NGT	0.2 (1.64)	1.6 (1.00)	0.4 (1.92)	32.4 (2.01)

*The units are volts per meter and milliamps per meter.

[†]p < 0.05 for the difference between VDT (IBM and CCI units combined) and non-VDT units (LED and NGT units).

change with increasing distance from the unit. These data indicated that the electrical environment in the room contributed to the ELF exposure of the general operators, rather than the LED unit with which they were working.

QUESTION 14. Based upon Table 1.4, what other analysis might be done to evaluate the risk of SAB for VDT users?

While NIOSH investigators were completing this research, six other studies of spontaneous abortion in relation to VDT use were published (Ericson and Kallen, 1986; Bryant and Love, 1989; Nielsen and Brandt, 1990; Windham et al., 1990; McDonald et al., 1988; Goldhaber et al., 1988). These studies utilized interview information or description of job duties to estimate VDT use. One was intended to evaluate the potential contribution of physical and psychological stress (Nielsen and Brandt, 1990). None of the studies measured the electromagnetic fields. Four of these studies were negative (Ericson and Kallen, 1986; Bryant and Love, 1989; Nielsen and Brandt, 1990; Windham et al., 1990), one was positive (Goldhaber et al., 1988), and another was positive using an interview definition of VDT use and negative using a definition of VDT use based upon job duties (McDonald et al., 1988). At the writing of this exercise, the bulk of the research indicates that VDT technology does not pose a risk for miscarriage. The results of studies now underway should help resolve this question.

References

Berquist U: Video display terminals and health: a technical and medical appraisal of the state of the art. Scand J Work Environ Health 10 (Suppl 2):62–67, 1984.

Bryant H, Love E: Video display terminal use and spontaneous abortion risk. Int J Epidemiol 18:132–38, 1989.

Goldhaber M, Polen M, Hiatt R: The risk of miscarriage and birth defects among women who use visual display terminals during pregnancy. Am J Indust Med 13:695–706, 1988.

Ericson A, Kallen B: An epidemiological study of work with video screens and pregnancy outcome: I. A registry study. Am J Indust Med 9:447–57, 1986.

Mamelle N, Laumon B, Lazar P: Prematurity and occupational activity during pregnancy. Am J Epidemiol 119:309–322, 1984.

Mausner J, Baun A: Epidemiology—An Introductory Text. Philadelphia: W.B. Saunders Company, 1974.

McDonald A, McDonald J, Armstrong B, et al.: Work with visual display units in pregnancy. Br J Indust Med 45:509–15, 1988.

Naeye R, Peters E: Working during pregnancy: effects on the fetus. Pediatrics 69:724–727, 1982.

Nielsen C, Brandt L: Spontaneous abortion among women using video display terminals. Scand J Work Environ Health 16:323–28, 1990.

Schnorr T, Grajewski B, Hornung R, et al.: Video display terminals and the risk of spontaneous abortion. New Engl J Med 324:727–33, 1991.

Tell R: An investigation of electric and magnetic fields and operator exposures produced by VDT's. NIOSH VDT epidemiology study, final report, NIOSH, Cincinnati, Ohio (NTIS publication no., PB 91-13-500), 1990.

Windham G, Fenster L, Swan S, et al.: Use of video display terminals during pregnancy and the risk of spontaneous abortion, low birthweight, or intrauterine growth retardation. Am J Indust Med 18:675–88, 1990.

ANSWERS

ANSWER 1. Ideally, spontaneous abortions might be identified from a record-based data source. However, these sources are not easily available in the United States, and those that are available contain only late (> 8–10 weeks gestation) spontaneous abortions. In practice this meant that a case-control study of spontaneous abortion was not possible. Researchers chose instead a cohort design. This too was attractive, because multiple reproductive outcomes could be observed. While the principal outcome of interest was spontaneous abortion, investigators also wanted to observe other outcomes.

A group of married women exposed to VDTs and not exposed to VDTs during a fixed period would be studied. A retrospective study of pregnancies over a limited period of time among exposed and nonexposed women would be the quickest approach, but might involve the usual problems of retrospective studies concerning accurate assessment of reproductive outcome and ascertainment of amount (e.g., hours per week) of VDT exposure. A prospective study might overcome these problems but take longer. Also, a prospective study might not be feasible due to rapid changes in the exposure status of the study population, since changes in office technology were occurring at a rapid pace.

Researchers chose a retrospective design with the option of later continuing with a prospective study of the same population. It was decided to use a telephone interview to identify the reproductive outcome of the pregnancies and then to attempt to verify this information from birth certificates and medical records. Amount of VDT "exposure" was to be determined, if possible, from company records as well as the interviews.

ANSWER 2. Researchers chose "VDT use" as the principal exposure variable. VDT use had been the focus of public concern, and researchers wanted to compare spontaneous abortion risk among VDT users to the risk among women who did not use VDTs. Level of exposure was to be determined by frequency of VDT use (hours per week during pregnancy).

While researchers could not be sure which if any of the three hypothesized exposures associated with VDTs (electromagnetic radiation, physical stress, psychological stress) was most important, they focused on electromagnetic radiation given off by the VDT as the most plausible exposure that might be associated with spontaneous abortions. They planned to measure such radiation among a representative sample of VDT users and non–VDT users.

Psychological and physical stress are hard to define and come from many sources, making it difficult to control for these possible risk factors. The investigators decided to "match" on these factors by choosing a study population in which both exposed and nonexposed groups would share the same level of psychologic and physical stress. Hence, any difference in abortion rate between VDT users and nonusers would be due to the remaining factors such as electromagnetic fields.

ANSWER 3. Sample size calculations prior to beginning a study are somewhat more complicated for a cohort study of reproductive outcomes than for other types of cohort study. The unit of observation in the study was a pregnancy. Women who did not become pregnant during the study period could not enter the study (e.g., those using birth control). However, determining sample size for the study did require determining the number of women who would have the needed number of pregnancies. Investigators decided a priori that they wanted to be able to detect a relative risk of 1.5 with 90% power, assuming an alpha level of 0.05. Calculations involved cumulative incidence or count data because the risk period was short and most people would have the same follow-up time, permitting the calculation of meaningful relative risks without the use of person-year data.

Researchers used published data on birth rates of married and working women to estimate sample size (e.g., NCHS 1982). The birth rate estimates based on a variety of sources were approximately the same. The rates ranged from 69.3 births/1,000 women when *all* working, married women were considered, to 206 births/1,000 women when only women aged 15–24 (in 1972) were considered. It therefore seemed reasonable to assume a rate of 100 births/1,000 working, married women for sample-size estimations. The follow-up period was defined as 1/83–12/86, a period short enough so that women could recall well any abortions but long enough to allow for one or more births per married woman. Two companies where the study would take place were tentatively identified.

To be eligible for the study, women had to have been pregnant while employed. It was known from company data that the average length of employment for women potentially eligible for the study was only 1.7 years. Investigators assumed a birth rate of 100 births/1,000 working, married women/year. They also assumed a 15% spontaneous abortion rate. They then derived the following sample size and power estimates (the sample sizes below apply to a single group, either exposed or nonexposed):

Outcome	Detectable Rel Risk	No. Married, Employed Women	No. Live Births	No. Pregnancies
Spontaneous	1.5	2,835	482	567
abortion	1.6	2,025	344	405
	2.0	806	137	167

Approximately 2,835 married, employed women were needed in both the exposed and referent groups in order to detect a 1.5-fold increase in spontaneous abortions with 90% power.

ANSWER 4. Important potential confounders in such a study are factors known to be associated with spontaneous abortions and possibly associated with exposure (Kline et al., 1989; Potter 1980). These include: medical conditions (including diabetes, thyroid conditions, epilepsy, cancer, and heart), prior induced abortion, prior spontaneous abortion, medications (including tranquilizers, sedatives, antinausea medications), X rays, infectious diseases, parity, alcohol consumption, smoking, and age.

ANSWER 5. Approximately half of the women with missing phone numbers were currently employed by the phone companies. A NIOSH staff member called the women at work, obtained their home phone numbers, and arranged times for interviews. Because operators were generally not allowed to receive calls at work, this required some coordination with the company.

For operators who were no longer employed at the study companies, the tracing task was more difficult. For these women, those residing in nine large metropolitan areas were identified (about 26% of the former operators had moved to another region of the country or resided outside the major metropolitan areas). NIOSH then sent a trained field interviewer to the woman's home, requested her home phone number, and arranged a time for a telephone interview.

ANSWER 6. In the analysis of spontaneous abortions (SAB), researchers defined an SAB as any fetal loss ≤28 weeks gestation. (SAB is sometimes defined as ≤20 weeks, as well.) Pregnancies ending in induced abortions were not at risk of spontaneous abortion, and were excluded from the analysis. Similarly, ectopic pregnancies are not implanted in the womb, and generally cannot result in a live birth or spontaneous abortion. These were also excluded from the analysis. Twin pregnancies are at increased risk of spontaneous abortion, and it is not uncommon for the twins to have different outcomes (e.g., spontaneous abortion, live birth). Investigators chose to include such pregnancies and consider a twin pregnancy as a risk factor in the analysis.

ANSWER 7. The crude SAB rates are merely the number of SABs in the group divided by the number of SABs and live births.

	Unexposed Pregnancies	*Exposed Pregnancies*
Crude SAB rate:	82/516 = 15.9%	54/366 = 14.8%

The relative risk is then the ratio of these two rates:

Crude Relative Risk = 14.8% / 15.9% = 0.93

The SAB rate by month of gestation must be calculated using the number of pregnancies at risk as the denominator. Thus, the SABs in the previous month must be subtracted from the denominator in the subsequent month. The four SABs for which the month of gestation was unknown were omitted.

Spontaneous Abortion Rate by Month of Gestation

Month of Gestation	*Unexposed Pregnancies, No. SABs/No. Pregnancies ·at risk = rate (%)*	*Exposed Pregnancies, No. SABs/No. Pregnancies at risk = rate (%)*
1	10/512 = 2.0%	1/366 = 0.3%
2	38/502 = 7.5	30/365 = 8.2
3	15/462 = 3.2	12/335 = 3.6
4	7/449 = 1.6	5/323 = 1.5
5	2/442 = 0.5	4/318 = 1.3
6	4/440 = 0.9	1/314 = 0.3
7	2/436 = 0.5	1/313 = 0.3

These initial findings did not indicate any pronounced difference in SAB rate between exposed and nonexposed women, either for the entire pregnancy or by month of gestation.

ANSWER 8. The Mantel-Haenszel point estimate for the risk ratio stratified by smoking status and prior abortion is 0.90. The chi-square test of overall association is 0.42, resulting in a test-based confidence interval of 0.66–1.23.

ANSWER 9. The relative risks are 1.17 and .92, respectively, indicating no trend. The chi-square test for trend is 0.08 (p = .78).

ANSWER 10. Logistic regression results for the odds ratio of VDT exposure during the first trimester (13 weeks), controlling for smoking (yes or no) and prior abortion, are 0.88, which compares well with the Mantel-Haenszel estimate of the risk ratio of 0.90. A prior thyroid condition is a significant predictor of SAB. Smoking as a continuous variable is a better predictor than simply using smoking as a yes/no variable. A model with smoking as a continuous variable, prior spontaneous abortion, prior thyroid condition, and average hours of VDT use during the first trimester shows that the number of cigarettes smoked exhibits a dose response with the risk of SAB, but that the number of hours of VDT use does not. No interactions are important.

ANSWER 11. The simplest method that could be used would be to limit the analysis to one pregnancy per woman (e.g., the first). This is the method that had been employed by researchers in the past, and when used here there was no change in results. New statistical techniques have been developed to allow for analysis of correlated outcomes (Zeger and Liang, 1986), but these also did not change results.

ANSWER 12. Differences in the rate or timing of induced abortions between the exposed and comparison groups might affect the results. For example, if the exposed groups had more induced abortions or had them earlier in gestation, then those pregnancies would not be at risk of spontaneously aborting. The exposed group could, therefore, show an artificially reduced risk of spontaneous abortion. Investigators looked at the rate and timing of induced abortions and found that VDT-exposed pregnancies had a rate of 4.8% and unexposed pregnancies had a rate of 5.3%. Gestational age at the time of the induced abortion was not markedly different between the two groups (mean number of weeks at abortion 9.6 and 7.9, respectively).

ANSWER 13. Investigators looked at the validity of reports of spontaneous abortion by examining the birth certificates of live births for those women who reported live births following a SAB. The women who reported 77 (38%) of the 203 spontaneous abortions between 1983 and 1986 had subsequent live births. It was found that 89% (49 of 55) of the SABs reported by the general operators and 86% (19 of 22) of the spontaneous abortions reported by directory assistance operators were recorded on subsequent birth certificates. Although investigators were able to review only those spontaneous abortions that were followed by a live birth, the birth certificate analysis generally confirmed self-reported SABs for both VDT users and nonusers, with no pronounced overreporting by either group.

ANSWER 14. Because the electromagnetic field measurements were higher for the CCI model compared to the IBM model, additional analyses were conducted that included separate exposure variables for pregnancies during which the women used CCI or IBM units. No difference was found in the risk of spontaneous abortion between women using the CCI unit (OR = 0.92; 95% CI 0.58–1.47) and those using an IBM unit (OR = 0.98; 95% CI 0.58–1.64).

References for Answers

Kline J, Stein Z, Susser M: *Conception to Birth: Epidemiology of Prenatal Development,* Vol. 14 of Monographs in Epidemiology and Biostatistics. New York: Oxford University Press, 1989.

NCHS, Working women and childbearing: US, Vital and Health Statistics, Department of Health and Human Services, PHS 82-1985, Hyattsville, Maryland, 1982.

Potter J: Hypothyroidism and reproductive failure. Surg Gynecol Obstet 50:251–255, 1980.

Zeger SL, Liang K-Y: Longitudinal data analysis for discrete and continuous outcomes. Biometrics 42:121–130, 1986.

Chapter 2

Heart Disease Mortality among Workers Exposed to Carbon Monoxide in New York City

FRANK STERN AND KYLE STEENLAND

Carbon monoxide (CO) contributes to cardiovascular disease through several accepted and potential mechanisms, including binding to hemoglobin and reducing oxygen dissociation at the tissue level by shifting the oxygen-hemoglobin dissociation curve. Such oxygen deprivation may contribute to heart attacks, particularly in individuals whose hearts already are weakened by subclinical cardiovascular disease. Several experimental human studies of CO have focused on the acute effects on the heart of high-level CO exposure (for example, see Allred et al., 1989), but tens of thousands of workers are exposed to chronic low levels. NIOSH investigators wished to study the effects of long-term chronic exposure to CO. The target population were traffic control officers: (1) stationed in toll facilities on bridges, and (2) employed in observation booths within the tunnels. Industrial hygiene surveys in the 1960s showed that officers on bridges at that time were exposed to an average carbon monoxide concentration of about 13 parts per million (ppm), while officers in tunnels were exposed to an average carbon monoxide concentration of 51 ppm.

QUESTION 1. What type of study could be done to best evaluate cardiovascular mortality?

QUESTION 2. What are the major advantages and limitations to this type of study?

Materials and Methods

NIOSH investigators decided to conduct an historical cohort mortality investigation of the bridge and tunnel cohort. Workers had to be employed for at least one day between January 1, 1952, and February 10, 1981, to be included. Follow-up for vital status would extend through 1981.

QUESTION 3. What sources of follow-up could be used to determine the vital status of the cohort members?

Investigators decided to use the United States population from 1940 to 1984 and New York City population from 1950 to 1984 as the nonexposed comparison populations.

QUESTION 4. Why would New York City mortality rates be more useful for this study as comparison rates than the U.S. mortality rates?

QUESTION 5. Comparison rates from a working population are especially useful for occupational cohort studies. Why are they useful? Why would they be particularly useful in this study? Can you think of an appropriate worker comparison population for this study?

In the analyses of the cohort, a modified life table analysis system (Steenland et al., 1990) was initially used to compute expected number of deaths based upon person-years at risk and the New York City population death rates, and standardized mortality ratios (SMRs) were obtained for various causes of death.

QUESTION 6. What are the limitations of the SMR analyses used here? What type of additional analysis could be used?

Results

Table 2.1 shows the vital status of the study population, for bridge and tunnel officers. Complete study results can be found in Stern et al. (1988). As can be seen, a 97% follow-up rate was achieved for both groups. The percentage of tunnel officers who died (13%) was almost twice that of bridge officers (7%).

QUESTION 7. Do the above data indicate that the death rate of tunnel officers is about twice that of bridge officers?

In the 30-year period between January 1, 1952, and January 1, 1982, the overall mortality among bridge officers was less than expected: 314 deaths observed vs. 409.0 expected, SMR = 0.76, when compared to the mortality of the New York City population. The SMR for heart disease was 0.84 (85% CI 0.71–0.99). The overall mortality among tunnel officers was slightly greater than expected: 160 deaths observed compared with 153 expected, SMR = 1.04. The SMR for heart disease for tunnel officers was 1.24 (95% CI 1.01–1.51). Heart disease mortality for tunnel officers was particularly high for

TABLE 2.1 Vital Status (as of 1982) and Demographic Characteristics
of Male Bridge and Tunnel Officers

Vital Status	Bridge Officers	Tunnel Officers	Total
Alive	3,872 (90%)	1,014 (84%)	4,886 (88%)
Deceased	314 (7%)	160 (13%)	474 (9%)
With death certificates	303	157	460
Without death certificates	11	3	14
Lost to follow-up	131 (3%)	38 (3%)	169 (3%)
Total	4,317	1,212	5,529
Person-years at risk	79,865	24,035	103,900
Year of Birth (mean)	1936	1930	
% white	83	80	
Year first employed (mean)	1963	1961	

arteriosclerotic heart disease (ASHD) (SMR = 1.35, 95% CI 1.09–1.68, 61 obs. vs. 45 exp.). After ten years of employment for tunnel officers, the mortality from ASHD increased to 88% over expected (SMR = 1.88, 95% CI 1.36–2.56, 30 obs. vs. 16 exp.). No such increasing trend was observed for bridge officers.

QUESTION 8. How accurate do you think death certificates are for heart disease? How would such inaccuracy affect study results?

To illustrate how expected deaths are calculated in an SMR analysis, the following data represent five tunnel officers:

Tunnel Officer	Age Started Work	Year Started Work	Year Stopped Work	Death Year (if died)
	(assume Jan. 1 date of birth)	(assume Jan. 1)	(assume Dec. 31)	(assume Dec. 31)
A	30	1955	1957	
B	20	1962	1974	
C	26	1955	1974	1976
D	21	1937	1977	
E	17	1941	1954	1968

Assume that there were no breaks between the first and last dates employed. Note that because of Jan. 1 birth dates, worker A just became 30 years of age on the day he started work, Jan. 1, 1955.

QUESTION 9. Calculate the person-years at risk for each combination of age, calendar time, and length of employment in the cells below (thanks to James Beaumont for the original development of this question). Accompany each entry with the corresponding identifying letter (e.g., if A contributed five person-years to the top left cell, enter "A = 5". (Hint: Workers D and E started work before 1952 but did not contribute person-years at risk until 1952, because work in 1952 or later was a study criterion. If they had contributed person-years before 1952 they would have been "immortal." This is because it was necessary for them to survive until 1952 in order to enter the study. In this study it was impossible to have deaths prior to 1952, and therefore the years before 1952 were not "at risk."

Employment 0–9 Yr
Calendar Time

Age	50–59	60–69	70–79	80–81
20–39	A = 5			
40–59				
60+				

Employment 10+ Yr
Calendar Time

Age	50–59	60–69	70–79	80–81
20–39				
40–59				
60+				

QUESTION 10. Assume that the death rates for the population over the study period have been as follows:

Age	1950–59	1960–69	1970–79	1980–81
20–39	.002	.001	.001	.001
40–59	.05	.02	.01	.003
60+	.4	.3	.25	.1

Using the cells below, what are the expected and observed number of deaths in each cell? What is the total number of expected deaths? What is the SMR?

Employment 0–9 Yr
Calendar Time

Age	50–59	60–69	70–79	80–81
20–39				
40–59				
60+				

Employment 10+ Yr
Calendar Time

Age	50–59	60–69	70–79	80–81
20–39				
40–59				
60+				

TABLE 2.2 Trend in Heart Disease Death for Tunnel Officers by Duration of Employment

| | Duration Employed (years) | | |
	<5	5–10	10+
Observed	27	4	30
Expected	25.6	3.4	15.9
SMR	105	118	189

QUESTION 11. Suppose an additional entry criterion was having to work for at least three years. What year would worker A, B, C, D, and E start contributing person-years?

QUESTION 12. In the actual data there was an apparent trend in ASHD with duration of employment for tunnel workers, with SMRs for <10, 10–20, and 20+ years employment, (see Table 2.2). Use the Breslow et al. test described in the Appendix to test whether this apparent trend was statistically significant (assume category midpoints of 2.5, 7.5, and 15 year of employment). How would you interpret this trend?

QUESTION 13. A direct comparison between bridge and tunnel workers was done using direct standardization with the data shown below in Table 2.3 (the weights were the combined person-years of both groups). Calculate the directly standardized rate ratio. Comment on the result compared to the SMR result of a 35% excess risk of heart disease compared to New York City population (especially in light of your response to Question 5.

TABLE 2.3 Deaths and Person-Years for Tunnel and Bridge Officers

Age	Calendar Time	Tunnel Officers		Bridge Officers	
		Observed Deaths	Person Years	Observed Deaths	Person-Years
<50	<1970	7	10697	17	32598
50+	<1970	3	715	2	1462
<50	1970–74	5	3349	9	13594
50+	1970–74	18	1157	13	1998
<50	1975+	3	4560	14	22723
50+	1975+	25	3550	34	7500

TABLE 2.4 Rate Ratios* (90% confidence intervals) for Heart Disease Mortality, by Time Since Last Date of Employment and by Age at Death, among Male Tunnel Officers Relative to Male Bridge Officers

Age	*0–1 Month*	*2–23 Months*	*2–4 Years*	*≥5 Years*
		Time Since Last Date of Employment		
45	0.98	1.39	2.11	0.94
	(0.51–1.89)	(0.53–3.63)	(0.68–6.58)	(0.59–1.50)
55	1.59	2.25	3.41†	1.51
	(0.85–2.95)	(0.88–5.76)	(1.11–10.43)	(0.99–2.30)
65	2.57†	3.63†	5.53‡	2.45†
	(1.18–5.58)	(1.27–10.34)	(1.65–18.56)	(1.31–4.58)

*Estimated using the Cox proportional hazards model.
†Significantly different from 1.00 ($p < 0.05$).
‡Significantly different from 1.00 ($p < 0.01$).

Tunnel workers were also compared directly to bridge workers for heart disease mortality by time-since-*last*-employment (see Table 2.4), using a Cox regression model.

QUESTION 14. Can you explain why heart disease mortality rates would increase initially after cessation of employment for any workers? Can you explain why this increase would be even more pronounced for those with higher CO exposure? Are the data in Table 2.4 consistent with such a phenomenon?

In 1970, the Triborough Bridge and Tunnel Authority added fresh ventilation in all tunnel tollbooths, along with a 15% increase in tunnel ventilation. To investigate what effect that had on ASHD mortality, trends in ASHD mortality after that time were evaluated. A significant decrease in the heart disease mortality death rate was found ($p = 0.042$) after 1970 compared to before 1970, using a regression model.

Discussion

This investigation was the first that studied the mortality effects of occupational exposures to carbon monoxide. Results indicated that there was an association between an exposure (carbon monoxide) and a disease (arteriosclerotic heart disease).

QUESTION 15. Do the results indicate that the association (between carbon monoxide and heart disease) is causal (i.e., exposure to carbon monoxide causes heart disease)? What criteria can be evaluated to assess causality?

References

Allred E, Bleecker E, Chaitman B, et al.: Short-term effects of carbon monoxide exposure on the exercise performance of subjects with coronary artery disease. New Engl J Med 321:1426–1475, 1989.

Steenland et al.: New developments in the NIOSH life-table analysis system. JOM 32,11:1091–1098, 1990.

Stern F, Halperin W, Hornung R: Heart disease mortality among bridge and tunnel officers exposed to carbon monoxide. Am J Epidemiol 128,6:1276–1288, 1988.

ANSWERS

ANSWER 1. A mortality study of the target population could theoretically be done via a case-control study or a cohort study. A population-based case-control study, with cases being all heart disease deaths in New York City over some defined period, and controls being other deaths, would have had relatively low power because the prevalence of exposure (working as traffic control officer) would have been low. Ascertainment of exposure in such a study would have been difficult, and might have required the computerization of the cohort of traffic control officers to cross-check against the cases and controls chosen from the general population. Such computerization would have meant accomplishing the most difficult part of a record-based cohort study. A case-control study of heart disease nested within the target population was not possible without some method to determine who among these workers had died of heart disease over some fixed period of time. Ascertainment of fatal heart attacks would require vital status ascertainment of the whole cohort, equivalent to a retrospective cohort study. Due to these considerations, a retrospective cohort study was the design of choice. Death from heart disease is a common outcome, and a cohort study would be expected to have sufficient statistical power to detect any elevated risk. A retrospective cohort mortality study was chosen, and to lower costs it was decided that it should be record-based (no interviews).

ANSWER 2. Retrospective cohort studies can examine the mortality of workers from the past to the present, avoiding the lengthy follow-up of a prospective study. Vital status for a mortality study can be ascertained from records alone, with no interviews. A cohort approach meant that other outcomes besides heart disease could be studied. Not doing interviews meant the study was relatively inexpensive, but had the disadvantage of failing to gather data on risk factors for heart disease (smoking, obesity, blood pressure). Interviews for the entire cohort would have made possible not only the collection of data on these risk factors but also the study of nonfatal heart disease, but the study would have cost perhaps five to ten times as much. One possibility was to conduct a record-based cohort mortality study, and as a later phase conduct a nested case-control study in which the cases would be decedents who died of heart disease. Interviews with next of kin and medical records could then provide information on the principal risk factors for heart disease. NIOSH investigators chose to begin with the retrospective record-based cohort mortality study, with a decision on a subsequent nested case-control study postponed.

ANSWER 3. Various sources of follow-up can be used. If SSA numbers are available, the Social Security Administration (SSA) can be used to identify deaths from 1938 to present, assuming an individual was paying into the social security system. Another good source of follow-up, which was available to NIOSH investigators although not to the general public, is the Internal Revenue Service (IRS). Using SSA numbers, the IRS can determine whether an individual has recently paid taxes, and can also provide addresses. With an address an investigator can use the U.S. Postal Service. A postal inquiry can be sent to the U.S. Postal Service for each individual with the most recent address and the Postal Service will indicate if the individual is still living at that residence, has moved, or is recently deceased. Another excellent source of follow-up is the National Death Index (NDI), which keeps a depository of all deaths since 1979. NDI requires identifiers such as last name, date of birth, and/or social security number.

ANSWER 4. Rates from large populations, such as the general population of the United States, are often preferred because they are large enough to be stable. However, it is often better to use regional or state rates if rates for disease vary by region. New York City rates are large enough for stability and yet more clearly address geographical differences in mortality that may be caused by environmental conditions, differences in diet, smoking habits, etc.

ANSWER 5. Mortality rates from the general population include individuals who are often too sick to work. Occupational cohorts usually have mortality rates below expected, in comparison to a general population, when no occupational risk is present. This phenomenon, known as the "healthy worker effect," is characterized by a lower relative mortality from all causes combined, because relatively healthy individuals are likely to gain employment and remain employed.

For cardiovascular diseases, the healthy worker effect is stronger than for most other causes of death for two reasons. First, on initial hire, cardiovascular diseases can be readily detected so the potential employee is never hired. Second, blue-collar workers usually cannot suffer from heart disease and continue the physical activity required by their jobs; instead, they must leave employment. One method to avoid the healthy worker effect is to compare workers with other workers. In this case, more highly exposed tunnel officers were compared with less exposed bridge officers.

ANSWER 6. Two limitations of any life table analysis with SMRs are: (1) continuous variables (such as duration of employment, age, latency, and calendar time) must be categorized, with data grouped into strata, causing some loss of precision in the analysis; (2) indirect standardization (the SMR method) may make it invalid to compare subgroups of the exposed with each other. In addition, in the SMR analysis used here, in which the New York City population is the referent group, the tunnel and bridge workers would both be expected to have relatively low heart disease mortality due to the healthy worker effect.

There are other alternative methods of analysis that can be used. As mentioned above, a direct comparison of tunnel and bridge workers was possible, which would eliminate the problem of the healthy worker effect. This comparison could be done via life table methods (but using direct standardization), or by use of a regression model (e.g., Cox regression). A regression model permits the simultaneous adjustment for several confounder variables, (e.g., race, age, and calendar time), assessment of effect modifications (interaction, e.g., between age and exposure), and the use of continuous exposure variables (e.g., duration of exposure).

ANSWER 7. Although tunnel officers seem to have an almost twofold crude risk of death over that of bridge officers, various potentially confounding characteristics have not been considered at this point. For example, one must take into account the age distributions of the two groups to determine if the death rates are comparable. Table 2.1 shows that tunnel officers were older.

ANSWER 8. Only limited data exist on this issue. One report used the autopsy as the "gold standard" to assess the validity of death certificate data (Kirscher et al., 1985). The predictive value of death certificate diagnosis (rate of confirmation by autopsy data) was 79% for all circulatory disease (cancer had the best confirmation rate, 88%). Specific data for arteriosclerotic heart disease were not given in this report. The overall point is that there is some, but not major, misclassification of disease status for heart disease on death certificates. As long as this misclassification is equal for exposed and nonexposed, the net result will be a relatively small bias of the rate ratio toward the null value (1.00).

ANSWER 9.

Age	Employment 0–9 Yr Calendar Time				Employment 10+ Yr Calendar Time			
	50–59	60–69	70–79	80–81	50–59	60–69	70–79	80–81
20–39	A = 5 C = 5	A = 5 B = 8 C = 5	B = 2		D = 4 E = 8	C = 4 E = 4	B = 8	B = 2
40–59		A = 5	A = 10	A = 2	D = 4	C = 1 D = 10 E = 4	C = 6 D = 6	
60+							D = 4	D = 2
Total	10	23	12	2	16	23	25	4	115

ANSWER 10.

Age	Employment 0–9 Yr Calendar Time				Employment 10+ Yr Calendar Time			
	50–59	60–69	70–79	80–81	50–59	60–69	70–79	80–81
20–39	*O = 0 *E = .020	O = 0 E = .018	O = 0 E = .002		O = 0 E = .024	O = 0 E = .008	O = 0 E = .008	O = 0 E = .002
40–59		O = 0 E = .100	O = 0 E = .100	O = 0 E = .006	O = 0 E = .200	O = 1 E = .300	O = 1 E = .120	
60+							O = 0 E = 1.0	O = 0 E = .200
Total	O = 0 E = .020	O = 0 E = .118	O = 0 E = .102	O = 0 E = .006	O = 0 E = .224	O = 1 E = .308	0 = 1 E = 1.128	O = 0 E = .202	O = 2 E = 2.108

*O = Observed deaths; E = expected deaths.

The total number of expected deaths = 2.108.
The total number of observed deaths = 2.
The SMR = 2/2.108 = 0.95.

ANSWER 11.

Worker	A	1958
	B	1965
	C	1958
	D	1952
	E	1952

ANSWER 12. The chi-square test for trend in SMRs over duration of employment yields a chi-square (one degree of freedom) of 10381/(5338 − 3255) = 4.98, and the p-value is 0.026. This trend for many substances might indicate an increased risk with increased dose, if duration were a good surrogate for cumulative dose. In the case of CO, however, it may not be cumulative dose that is of interest, because the effect on the heart may be acute, due to a short-term increase in carboxyhemoglobin. On the other hand, it might be that those with more duration of employment have simply had more incidents of intense exposure with increased carboxyhemoglobin, and that these incidents have had a cumulative damaging effect on the heart.

ANSWER 13. The directly standardized rate ratio is calculated using the combined person-years for the age and calendar-time specific rates, and then calculating a weighted average of the age- and calendar-time-specific rates separately for tunnel and bridge workers. The weighted rate for tunnel workers is 199.8/100,000, while the weighted rate for bridge workers is 119.5/100,000. The directly standardized rate ratio is 199.8/119.5 = 1.67. This rate ratio is higher than the SMR of the 1.35 comparing the tunnel workers to the New York City population. This is probably because the direct comparison of tunnel to bridge workers does not suffer from the healthy worker effect, which causes an artificially low rate ratio when tunnel workers are compared to the general population.

ANSWER 14. When workers get so sick that they can no longer work, they are often told by their physicians to retire or quit or to go on disability retirement. Soon after retirement or termination, they may succumb to their illness, producing an initial high mortality rate shortly after employment (see Steenland and Stayner, 1991). Hence bridge and tunnel workers alike would be expected to experience high mortality rates from heart disease shortly after they left employment. Because we hypothesized that CO might have an acute effect on the heart (causing a heart attack), we expected to see this same phenomenon (initial high mortality after employment), but we expected it might be even more pronounced in tunnel workers with high CO exposure than in bridge workers with low CO exposure. This interpretation is consistent with the data in Table 2.4 in that the *ratio* of heart disease mortality rates between tunnel and bridge workers is highest in the first four years after leaving work and then goes down. The rate ratios in Table 2.4 are stratified by age because the Cox model indicated an interaction between exposure (tunnel vs. bridge) and age.

ANSWER 15. This subject is a critical one for epidemiology. Much has been written about it. Without entering into more philosophical or statistical definitions of causality (for example, see Rothman, 1986), epidemiologists often use some criteria for causality that were originally proposed by Hill (1965), and that are presented below in somewhat modified (reduced) form.

STRENGTH OF THE ASSOCIATION. *The greater the relative risk, the more likely the factor is causally related to the outcome.*

In the current study, an overall relative risk 35% greater than expected was observed in comparing tunnel workers to the U.S. population. In a direct comparison to bridge workers, the excess risk was 67%. These are rather substantial excess risks for heart disease, and were based on relatively large numbers of deaths.

DOSE-RESPONSE RELATIONSHIPS. *If the risk of disease increases with the degree of exposure and/or length of employment, it is more likely the association is causal.*

The comparisons of tunnel workers with bridge workers or with a nonexposed (New York City) population did show that the tunnel workers (high exposure) had higher response (more disease) than two groups with lower or background exposures. However, in this analysis there were no data on exposure level (or dose) for each individual, so a more definitive evaluation of a dose-response was not possible (further work is now underway to try to estimate exposures for each individual in the study and to evaluate dose-response). On the other hand, there were some indications that increased exposure did lead to increased disease. Workers exposed before 1970, when ventilation was worse and exposures presumably higher, had more risk than those first exposed after 1970. The rate ratio for tunnel workers with longer duration was also increased. While the postulated effect of CO on the heart is acute, it is possible that longer-duration workers simply had repeated exposures to high level of CO, with damage to the heart accumulating over time. The trend with duration may also mean that there is some unknown chronic effect (plaque formation?) of CO on the heart beyond the hypothesized acute effect due to oxygen deprivation.

CONSISTENCY OF THE ASSOCIATION. *The association found in one study should hold up in other populations with other study methods.*

In the case of carbon monoxide, no other long-term mortality studies exist. Further studies are needed. However, experimental human studies (e.g., Allred et al., 1989) tend to support the association. Also, in this study results were consistent for both referent groups, the New York City population and the bridge workers.

TEMPORAL CORRECT ASSOCIATION. *The exposure should precede the onset of disease and allow for a necessary period of induction.*

The exposure to CO did precede the heart disease in this study. The *postulated* induction period is short (acute effect, an increase of carboxy-hemoglobin, triggering heart disease). The observed trend of decreasing relative risk for tunnel versus bridge workers with increasing time since last employment does conform to a risk of heart disease while working, which forces the worker to quit work, and causes initial high mortality shortly after last employment.

BIOLOGICAL PLAUSIBILITY. *The ability of some biological mechanism to explain the association.*

The biological mechanism through which CO causes its damage is its ability to decrease the oxygen-carrying capacity of the blood, which has an affinity for CO 210 times that of oxygen. The heart responds to this increased need by increasing coronary blood flow, heart rate, and blood pressure, producing myocardial symptoms such as angina pectoris, ECG abnormalities, arrhythmia, and ischemia.

In summary, most of the criteria, with the exception of a dose-response criteria, are satisfied in this study, lending support to the view that the association is causal.

References for Answers

Allred E, Bleecker E, Chaitman B, et al.: Short-term effects of carbon monoxide exposure on the exercise performance of subjects with coronary artery disease. N Engl J Med 321:1426–1475, 1989.

Hill A: The environment and disease: association or causation. Proc Roy Soc Med 58:295–300, 1965.

Kirscher T, Nelson J, and Burdo H: The autopsy as a measure of accuracy of the death certificate. N Engl J Med 313,20:1263–1269, 1985.

Rothman K: *Modern Epidemiology.* Boston: Little, Brown, 1986.

Steenland K, Stayner L: The role of employment status in occupational cohort mortality studies. Epidemiol 2: 418–423, 1991.

Chapter 3

Larynx Cancer Incidence among Workers Exposed to Acid Mists

KYLE STEENLAND

In the mid-1980s, at the time this study began, three reports in the literature indicated that exposure to acid mists (mainly sulfuric acid) was associated with an increase of larynx cancer (Soskolne et al., 1984; Forastiere et al., 1988; Ahlborg et al., 1981). However, these reports were inconclusive for several reasons: they were based on very small numbers, they lacked control over smoking, or they included people whose exposure to acid mists was uncertain. Hence, further study was warranted. The hypothesis that acid mists led to larynx cancer of the upper respiratory tract was biologically plausible. Acid mists irritate the epithelial cells of the upper respiratory tract and conceivably could be carcinogens. No animal studies had been done.

Investigators at the National Institute for Occupational Safety and Health (NIOSH) began to search for an appropriate population to study. The leading candidate was an existing cohort of 1,156 men exposed to acid mists during the pickling of steel. This cohort had already been studied for mortality by NIOSH investigators (Beaumont et al., 1987). The 1,156 men had worked at three midwestern steel plants from the 1940s through the 1980s. Their average duration of work in the pickling area was nine years.

Thirty-two percent of the acid mist cohort had died by 1985. The mortality study results had shown an excess of lung cancer. Regarding larynx cancer, two deaths had been observed versus one expected.

Acid pickling is done to remove impurities, and in this cohort the primary acid used was sulfuric acid. Exposures to sulfuric acid had generally been below the OSHA standard of 1.0 mg/cubic meter, and had changed little over time. Industrial hygiene sampling data showed no other occupational exposures to known carcinogens, such as nickel or chromium. Men with any coke oven exposure, which might increase the risk of larynx cancer, had been excluded from the cohort.

QUESTION 1a. What are the drawbacks of a mortality study of larynx cancer?

QUESTION 1b. What study design could be used to study larynx cancer among these steelworkers? What would be the nonexposed comparison group?

QUESTION 1c. Would such a study be worthwhile? This question should be addressed from the standpoint of statistical power, of public health, and of scientific/biologic interest.

QUESTION 1d. What are the principal known causes of larynx cancer? How could these other causes (potential confounders) be "controlled"?

Materials and Methods

NIOSH investigators decided to conduct a cohort incidence study of the steel-workers. Follow-up would be conducted by mailed questionnaire, to either the cohort member himself or his next of kin. The questionnaire would ask about cancer incidence, polyps incidence (possibly also associated with exposure), smoking, and drinking. Two questionnaires would be mailed. If there were no response to the mailed questionnaires, phone calls would be made.

The medical records of all decedents would be sought as an additional source of information regarding larynx cancer incidence.

Medical confirmation of any self-reported larynx cancers would also be sought.

QUESTION 2. What sources could be used to locate cohort members or their next of kin (recall that NIOSH is a federal agency)?

QUESTION 3. What difficulties would you predict in tracing cohort members and/or for obtaining medical records for decedents?

Investigators determined that the most complete and oldest data on age-specific laryngeal cancer incidence existed for the state of Connecticut, which had rates from 1935 to 1979. New York had rates available exclusive of New York City from 1950 to 1972. There were no complete national rates, but national surveys had been done for a sample of the country during three National Cancer Surveys (1938, 1948, 1970) and during two later SEER (Surveillance, Epidemiology, and End Results) surveys (1973–1977, and 1978–1981). These various surveys generally covered about 10% of the U.S. population and were considered representative. None of the cancer incidence data were broken down by smoking habits.

QUESTION 4. Why is it important that comparison rates be age-specific and specific to particular calendar periods?

QUESTION 5. What problems would you anticipate in using these rates as nonexposed comparison rates for this study? Which would you use?

Investigators decided to use all three sets of comparison rates and calculate a range of results. Figure 3.1 shows the rates that were available. Lines have been drawn between the points, but actual rates were available only at the calendar times indicated by the points. Figure 3.1 shows that Connecticut rates were highest for the period from 1960 on, while New York rates were lowest. Given that the points in Figure 3.1 for the respective locations appear to increase more or less linearly over time, investigators used simple linear regression to determine a best-fitting line for rates over time. For example, rates for 1949 to 1969 in the United States were determined using this regression procedure, since existing data were limited to 1948 and 1970 (in actuality, separate regressions were run for each set of age-specific rates).

The next problem was the method of control over smoking and drinking. Smoking and drinking habits of the cohort were known from the questionnaires, and smoking- and drinking-specific laryngeal cancer rates could be calculated. However, analogous smoking and drinking-specific laryngeal cancer rates were not available for any of the comparison populations. If they had been available, they would have allowed good control over confounding via

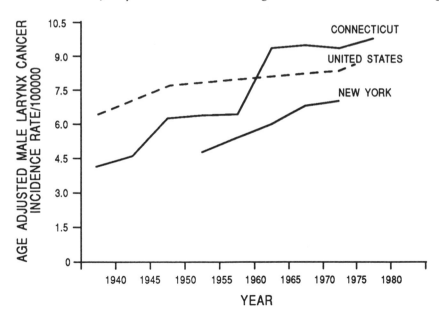

FIGURE 3.1 Age-adjusted incidence rates of male laryngeal cancer per 100,000 (adjusted to 1970 United States population).

stratification (the same technique used for age and calendar time). Exposed smokers would have been compared to nonexposed smokers, exposed nonsmokers to nonexposed nonsmokers, etc., and then a weighted average of these rate ratios would have been calculated.

Lacking such data, however, investigators needed other methods. There *were* some data on the smoking and drinking habits of the U.S. population at various times. Investigators decided to use an adjustment, known as the Axelson adjustment, to try to determine the effects of differing smoking and drinking habits between the exposed and nonexposed (Axelson, 1978). Inspection of the smoking and drinking habits of the exposed versus the nonexposed allowed the investigators to determine if they differed. If they did not differ, then smoking and drinking would not act as confounders and would not need to be controlled in the analysis. Suppose, however, they did differ. Suppose the exposed population smoked and drank more, for example, than did the comparison population. The Axelson technique would use the known effects of smoking and drinking on larynx cancer rates to predict how much difference in larynx cancer rates between exposed and nonexposed would be expected to occur due to smoking and drinking, under the assumption that there was no effect of exposure to acid mists whatsoever. Any difference in larynx cancer rates above and beyond those predicted by excess smoking and drinking by the exposed cohort might then be attributed to exposure to acid mists.

Results

Table 3.1 shows the questionnaire response rates for the study population. As expected, response rates for next of kin were worse than response rates for those still alive. The bulk of the nonresponse for the next of kin was due to the inability of the investigators to locate the next of kin, rather than refusal to complete the questionnaire.

QUESTION 6. In what ways could the level of nonresponse cause the study results to be invalid?

TABLE 3.1 Response Rate for Questionnaires

	Live	Next of Kin
Total sought	783	373
Completed interview	621 (79%)	220 (59%)
Mail interview	480	146
Telephone interview	141	74
Nonresponse	162 (21%)	153 (41%)
No address found	106	122
Some address found	56	31

Some medical record was obtained for 72% of the decedents, but only 45% of the decedents had medical records with adequate information to determine lifetime cancer incidence.

A decedent was allowed in the analysis if either the next of kin reported his cancer history or adequate medical record data were available. However, a larynx cancer reported by next of kin had to be confirmed by medical record to be accepted into the analysis.

Live individuals were admitted for analysis only if they had filled out a questionnaire or were interviewed by phone. No larynx cancers were accepted unless confirmed by a physician.

Altogether, 77% (n = 879) of the original cohort met these criteria and were eligible for the analysis of larynx cancer incidence. These men contributed over 27,000 person-years-at-risk of larynx cancer, with person-years-at-risk beginning at date of first exposure for each man (date of first working in pickling) and continuing until the date last observed (end of follow-up). For people who did not die and were successfully traced, the date last observed generally was sometime in 1986. For people who died, the date last observed was their date of death.

QUESTION 7. Would the criteria for admitting individuals into the analysis tend to increase or decrease larynx cancer rates among the exposed? Were these criteria relatively strict or liberal?

Table 3.2 shows the results for smoking data for the cohort and for the U.S. population, as of 1965 (1965 was chosen because smoking habits in the 1960s would be the most relevant for causing larynx cancers observed in the late 1970s or early 1980s, when most larynx cancers occurred in our cohort). Data on drinking are not presented here but showed the cohort and the U.S. population in general to have similar drinking habits.

QUESTION 8. Do the data in Table 3.2 indicate that the exposed cohort smoked more than the U.S. population sample? Smoking causes an approximate tenfold increase in larynx cancer rates (smokers versus nonsmokers). What would you guess would be the rate ratio of larynx

TABLE 3.2 Cigarette Smoking Data for the Cohort and the U.S. as of 1965

	Cohort	U.S. (age-adjusted)
Percentage never smoked cigarettes	24	24
Percentage current, 1 pack or less	34	40
Percentage current, more than 1 pack	27	15
Percentage former	15	21

cancer rates (exposed versus nonexposed) due to smoking differences alone?

Nine larynx cancers were observed in the cohort, five of whom had died. Only two of the decedents had any indication of larynx cancer on their death certificate. The nine cases averaged 26 years since first exposure, and averaged age 53 at diagnosis. All were smokers or former smokers.

To illustrate how expected deaths were calculated, Table 3.3 provides data on the person-years for the cohort in the period 1975–1979, as well as the estimated U.S. age-specific and calendar-time-specific larynx cancer rates. Data on the observed larynx cancers during this five-year period, by age at diagnosis, are also presented. For the actual overall calculation in the study, data similar to these were used, but covered the entire period from 1940 to 1986.

QUESTION 9. Calculate the overall expected number of larynx cancers during the 1975–1979 calendar period, based on the data in Table 3.3. Calculate the standardized rate ratio (observed to expected) during this period. For what variable (confounder) has this rate ratio been standardized? Is this an example of indirect or direct standardization? Show that the ratio of observed to expected is actually a ratio of two weighted averages of rates.

TABLE 3.3 Person-Years, Observed Larynx Cancers, and U.S. Comparison Larynx Cancer Rates (per 100,000)

Years	Age	Person-Years in Cohort	Observed Larynx Cancers	U.S. Rate
75–79	15–19	0	0	0.0
75–79	20–24	0	0	0.1
75–79	25–29	7	0	0.1
75–79	30–34	115	0	0.6
75–79	35–39	254	0	1.4
75–79	40–44	448	0	4.8
75–79	45–49	527	2	9.1
75–79	50–54	595	1	13.5
75–79	55–59	554	1	27.0
75–79	60–64	480	0	36.2
75–79	65–69	307	0	42.2
75–79	70–74	177	0	41.4
75–79	75–79	83	0	39.1
75–79	80–84	33	0	33.2
75–79	85+	6	0	23.5

For the entire study period (1940–1986), the overall expected larynx cancers, based on U.S., New York, and Connecticut rates, respectively, were 3.44, 2.94, and 3.89. Adjusting these expected figures upward 15% to account for excess smoking among the cohort, the expected larynx cancers were 3.92, 3.35, and 4.43, respectively, leading to standardized rate ratios of 2.30, 2.70, and 2.04, respectively.

QUESTION 10. Calculate the chi-square test of significance for the standardized rate ratio using U.S. rates as the reference rates. Is the rate ratio significantly different than 1.0? Calculate the test-based confidence intervals, or range of plausible values, for this same rate ratio.

Discussion

Regardless of which comparison population was used, this cohort experienced a twofold excess of larynx cancer, which was a statistically significant excess. Therefore, this study provides further evidence that exposure to acid mists is associated with larynx cancer. Although the numbers in this study were small, exposure were well characterized and an adjustment was made for smoking and drinking habits.

The fact that all the larynx cancers occurred among smokers or former smokers is not surprising, because virtually all larynx cancers in the general population also occur among smokers. Virtually no larynx cancers would have been expected to occur among the never-smokers in the cohort.

It is possible that acid mists acted as laryngeal carcinogens by facilitating the already strong carcinogenic effect of tobacco smoke.

About 75% of this cohort was exposed to sulfuric acid, and the remainder was largely exposed to hydrochloric acid. The data in our study were too sparse to be able to separate the effects of the different types of acid.

Among the live individuals in the study, nine men also reported benign growths on the vocal cords, one of which subsequently developed into larynx cancer. However, no expected numbers of such growths could be calculated because no standard rates were known, so it cannot be determined if these growths numbered more than might have been expected.

Further analyses were conducted by duration of exposure and time-since-first-exposure (potential latency), by dividing the person-years into less than five years exposure versus more than five years exposure, and less than 20 years since first exposure versus more than 20 years since first exposure. No clear differences were revealed between duration or potential latency groups with these analyses, which were based on small numbers.

QUESTION 11. Aside from the problem of imprecision, can an analysis of larynx cancer risk by duration of exposure be considered a kind of "dose-response" analysis? Can the lack of trend in the duration analysis in this study be taken as a lack of a dose-response?

References

Ahlborg G, Hogstedt C, Sundell L, et al.: Laryngeal cancer and pickling house vapors. Scand J Work Environ Health 7:239–240, 1981.

Axelson O: Aspects on confounding in occupational studies. Scand J Work Environ Health 4:85–89, 1978.

Beaumont J, Leveton J, Knox K, et al.: Lung cancer mortality in workers exposed to sulfuric acid mist and other acid mists in steel pickling operations. JNCI 79:911–921, 1987.

Forastiere F, Valesnin S, Salimei E, et al.: Respiratory cancer among soap production workers. Scand J Work Environ Health 13:258–260, 1987.

Soskolne C, Zeighami E, Hanis N, et al.: Laryngeal cancer and occupational exposure to sulfuric acid. Am J Epidemiol 120:358–369, 1984.

Steenland K, Schnorr T, Beaumont J, et al.: Incidence of laryngeal cancer and exposure to acid mists. J Indust Med 45:766–776, 1988.

ANSWERS

ANSWER 1a. Many people who have larynx cancer do not die of it. The five-year survival rate exceeds 50%. Hence, mortality is not a very sensitive outcome for larynx cancer, and incidence is to be preferred. The original mortality study had been conducted primarily to investigate lung cancer, which is usually fatal. Reports regarding larynx cancer and acid mists surfaced after the mortality study had been begun.

ANSWER 1b. A cohort incidence study was one possibility. One difficulty would be determining who among this cohort got larynx cancer. There are no central cancer registries in the United States (there are a number of statewide registries), which would have made possible a rapid identification of cases. Instead, each individual (or their next of kin) in the cohort would have to be contacted.

Another question was the choice of a nonexposed comparison group. There was no internal group of nonexposed individuals who could be used. The principal difficulty in using any external group would lie in determining their laryngeal cancer rates. There are several statewide cancer incidence registries that go back in time, and there are some data regarding national cancer incidence based on a sample of the U.S. population.

ANSWER 1c. Whether such a study would be worthwhile depends on two judgments, one mathematical and the other more subjective. The first question is whether the sample size of the study is large enough to answer the question posed: does exposure to acid mists cause larynx cancer? This involves a calculation of the "power" of the study to detect an excess risk of a specified size (the "power" to avoid a Type II error, the error of accepting the null hypothesis of no association when the alternative hypothesis is true). Let us assume from the prior studies that the postulated true relative risk for larynx cancer due to acid mist exposure is 2.0. A formula exists (Beaumont and Breslow, 1981) for calculating the power of a cohort study if the expected number of larynx cancers is known, and given a specified level of Type I error (the error of rejecting the null hypothesis when it is actually true, usually specificed as 5%). Generally, an 80% power is desired. Knowing the approximate number and age structure of the person-years at risk for this cohort from the already completed mortality study and knowing (at least approximately) the age-specific laryngeal cancer rates for a nonexposed population (see below), it was possible to determine that approximately three or four laryngeal cancers were expected. Using the formula cited above, the investigators determined that in this cohort there was sufficient power to detect a twofold risk of larynx cancer. From the standpoint of sample size the study appeared worthwhile.

The question of whether the study is worthwhile must also be addressed from the standpoint of public health. Larynx cancer is rare. However, it is a serious disease, often fatal, and substantial numbers of workers are exposed to acid mists. Furthermore, low-level exposure to acid mists is of concern for the general public due to acid rain. Following the cohort might also throw light on the previously observed excess of lung cancer mortality, a far more common disease.

From a scientific standpoint, the association of acid mists and larynx cancer was also of interest in that it might further elucidate possible mechanisms of carcinogenesis (e.g., acidic irritation of epithelial cells, leading to mutation, or inhibition of ciliary clearance mechanisms in the respiratory tract, leading to increased presence of other carcinogens such as cigarette smoke).

ANSWER 1d. The principal known causes of larynx cancer are smoking and drinking, with relative risks on the order of ten and two, respectively. These exposures could act as confounders, distorting the observed association between exposure and disease, if the exposed cohort and the nonexposed comparison group differed in their smoking and drinking habits. It would be necessary to control for these confounders (particularly smoking) by collecting information about them for both the exposed and nonexposed cohorts, and then somehow taking this information into account in the analysis.

ANSWER 2. The steelworker cohort had been assembled from personnel records at three steel plants. Names and Social Security numbers were known for each cohort member. NIOSH, as a federal agency, had access to Internal Revenue Service tax data regarding current addresses of those paying taxes, and these were used to locate live cohort members. Addresses from the death certificate were used to locate next of kin for the decedents. Directory assistance was used to obtain telephone numbers when addresses were not helpful.

ANSWER 3. Live individuals were relatively easy to trace, assuming they were paying taxes. It was much harder to trace the next of kin of dead individuals, especially if they had died long ago (deaths occurred from the 1950s to the 1980s). It was also difficult to obtain medical records for such men. NIOSH has legal rights to obtain medical records of decedents, and these were sought from the hospitals on the death certificates (most death certificates listed a hospital).

ANSWER 4. Larynx cancer rates have generally increased over time, largely due to increased smoking. Furthermore, larynx cancer rates, like most cancer rates, increase rapidly with age. Hence, age and calendar time were associated with disease and could act as potential confounders if exposed and nonexposed groups differed for these factors. To control for this possible confounding, data on larynx cancer incidence were to be stratified by age and calendar time. This would require age-specific and calendar-time-specific rates in both the exposed and nonexposed populations. Indirect standardization was used to create a summary rate ratio across age and calendar-time strata (see Question and Answer 9).

While age-specific rates were available both for the exposed cohort and the various possible comparison populations (Connecticut, New York, and the United States), the comparison populations did not consistently have rates available during the entire calendar period of interest (1940s through the 1980s). Some procedure would have to be adopted to confront this problem.

ANSWER 5. The exposed cohorts worked and lived in the Midwest, and it would have been preferable for the nonexposed comparison rates to come from the Midwest as well. It was not clear a priori whether Connecticut, New York, or the U.S. sample would provide the comparison group most similar to a nonexposed midwestern population, which was the ideal comparison group. Investigators decided to use all three sets of comparison rates and report a range of results.

ANSWER 6. The concern is that the nonrespondents might have had more or less larynx cancer than the respondents. There is no particular reason to believe that they did, and hence no real reason to suspect the population surveyed is not representative of the entire cohort. One could speculate that more larynx cancers may have occurred among decedents, who were underrepresented in the survey. If this were true, the survey population might have somewhat lower larynx cancer rates than the total cohort. Such a bias is called a "conservative" bias, and would only make a positive finding in the study more impressive.

ANSWER 7. The criteria were rather strict (conservative), and were more likely to have underestimated larynx cancer incidence than overestimated it. Next of kin, for example, who reported no cancer for the decedent may not have known about a larynx cancer, yet that person was admitted into the analysis. On the other hand, larynx cancers reported by next of kin were not admitted unless confirmed by medical record.

ANSWER 8. The data in Table 3.2 show that in 1965 the cohort and the United States had about the same percentage of never-smokers, but that among those who had ever smoked, there were fewer quitters among the cohort and more heavy current smokers. These data are typical of a blue-collar population versus the U.S. population. Since the early 1960s, blue-collar workers have smoked somewhat more than the general population. The Axelson adjustment discussed in the text, while not presented in detail here, predicted that larynx cancer rates among the exposed would be 15% higher than the U.S. population due to smoking differences (rate ratio of 1.15). The Axelson adjustment was also used to assess the effect of smoking differences as of 1976, and results were similar.

ANSWER 9. The overall expected (allow for some rounding error) is 0.73. There are three observed, and the standardized rate ratio is 4/.73, or 5.41. This rate ratio has been standardized for age. This is an example of indirect standardization. An indirectly standardized rate ratio is the ratio of two weighted averages of rates in which the weights used for both rates are the person-years of the exposed population. This is the same as the ratio of observed cancer cases to expected cases, as shown below:

$$
\frac{\dfrac{\sum_i w_i \times \text{rate}_{1i}}{\sum_i w_i}}{\dfrac{\sum_i w_i \times \text{rate}_{2i}}{\sum_i w_i}} = \frac{\sum_i w_i \times \text{rate}_{1i}}{\sum_i w_i \times \text{rate}_{2i}} =
$$

$$
\frac{\sum_i (\text{p-yr expos}_i) \times (\text{obsd cancers}_i/\text{p-yr expos}_i)}{\sum_i (\text{p-yr exps}_i) \times (\text{US rate}_i)} = \frac{\sum_i \text{obsd cancers}_i}{\sum_i \text{expd cancers}_i}
$$

ANSWER 10. Under the assumption that the observed is a Poisson variable with a mean equal to the expected, and based on the normal approximation to the Poisson distribution, the chi-square with one degree of freedom is

$$\chi_1^2 = \frac{(\text{observed} - \text{expected} - .05)^2}{\text{expected}} = \frac{(9 - 3.92 - .05)^2}{3.92} = 5.35$$

Consulting tables for the chi-square statistic with one degree of freedom, we find that the p-value for 5.35 is approximately 0.02, which means that the probability of finding nine or more observed cancers when only 3.92 were expected, if the null hypothesis of no exposure effect were true, was only 2%. Hence, we can reject the null hypothesis and find that the rate ratio is significantly elevated above the null rate ratio of 1.0. The 95% test-based confidence interval is $2.30^{(1 \pm 1.96/x)}$, or (1.13, 4.66).

The reader should note that more precise tests of significance and confidence limits are easily available via various software packages. We have used these approximations here because they are easily calculated by hand.

The above calculation treats the expected number of larynx cancers as invariant. Actually, due to the adjustment of the expected for smoking and drinking (15% increase), there is some variation associated with the expected number, which we have not considered here. This would tend to increase the width of the confidence interval for the rate ratio, although not dramatically.

ANSWER 11. Lack of an increasing cancer risk with increased duration of exposure should be considered with caution, and not necessarily be thought of as a lack of a dose-response. Duration is a crude surrogate for cumulative dose, especially in this case in which those with the highest doses were likely to have experienced the most irritation by the acid mists, and may have left the pickling job as a result.

References for Answers

Beaumont J, Breslow N: Power considerations in vinyl chloride studies. Am J Epidemiol 114:725–734, 1981.

Part II | Case-Control and Proportionate Mortality Studies

Case-control (or case-referent) studies begin with disease rather than exposure. The investigator chooses a group of individuals who have developed the disease of interest over a specific period of time (or died of the disease). He or she then also chooses a random sample of the nondiseased group from the same underlying population. For example, all bladder cancer cases occurring from 1980 to 1985 in the city of Cincinnati might form the case series, while a random sample of the population of Cincinnati who remained disease-free during that period might serve as controls. The exposure history of the cases and controls would then be compared to determine whether the cases are more likely to have been exposed than the controls.

The case-control study may be considered a variant of the cohort study. For example, suppose we enroll the entire population of Cincinnati in a ten-year study of bladder cancer incidence to determine whether smoking is associated with this type of cancer. Each person is interviewed to determine their smoking habits. At the end of ten years we determine the bladder cancer incidence rate in the smokers and compare it to the nonsmokers. If the smokers had more bladder cancer, we can conclude that smoking is associated with bladder cancer. Alternatively, without going through quite so much trouble, we may conduct a case-control study by identifying all those who developed bladder cancer in Cincinnati over the past ten years and then selecting a random sample of those who did not. Both groups may then be interviewed to determine the proportion of smokers. If the proportion of smokers is higher among the cases, we may conclude that smoking is associated with bladder cancer.

Depending on the situation, case-control studies can provide a less expensive and faster alternative to cohort studies. Case-control studies also have the advantage that the investigator can analyze the data for other exposures besides the one postulated a priori.

Case-control studies are particularly useful for rare diseases and for common exposures. A case series of a rare disease can be assembled by choosing all cases in a defined geographical area, for example. The exposure to be evaluated must be sufficiently common so that one might expect a significant proportion of cases and controls to be exposed. Otherwise, small numbers may impede the ability to detect an association. For example, a case-control study of end-stage renal disease and solvent exposure can be conducted by choosing all incident cases over a specified period of time from a statewide registry of all end-stage cases. Controls may then be selected from the general population of people who remained nondiseased over that period. The proportion of cases and controls exposed to solvents is likely to be appreciable, especially if the state is an industrial one in which solvent exposure in the workplace is common.

Case-control studies must ascertain exposure retrospectively, and this feature is a disadvantage compared to cohort studies. Exposure is often ascertained via interview, and study subjects may remember incorrectly their degree of exposure in the past. Hence, exposure status in cases and controls is quite often misclassified, which usually leads to a bias in the findings toward the null hypothesis if exposure is misclassified alike for cases and controls. Sometimes exposure is misclassified differentially—for example, if cases systematically overreport exposure. This can result if cases try harder to remember past exposures because they are searching for a cause for their disease. Such "recall bias" results in the proportion of exposed among the cases being artificially elevated compared to controls.

Case-control studies are only feasible when a case series can be assembled. Hence, they are done most easily for diseases that come to medical attention. It is important that both cases and controls be representative of the underlying population of interest (e.g., the city of Cincinnati). It is desirable that the cases represent all cases occurring in the population of interest, or at least a representative sample of them. Similarly, controls must represent the nondiseased population. It is particularly important that selection of cases and controls be done without any regard to their exposure status. Otherwise, a "selection bias" will result in which the exposure status of cases or controls will not be representative of the underlying population of interest.

Case-control studies are generally of three types: population-based, hospital-based, and nested within a cohort. The study of end-stage renal patients described above is an example of a population-based study, in which all new cases in the general population are chosen for study. Population-based controls may be randomly chosen from the nondiseased in the general population by a variety of methods, including random-digit dialing, using lists of those with driver's licenses, or choosing someone who lives next door to the index case. Population-based studies have the advantage that their results may be applicable to the entire general population in which the study was conducted.

Hospital-based case-control studies consist of a series of cases identified via a hospital or hospitals. Controls are chosen from the nondiseased in the same hospitals. Since the controls will have some other disease, special care must be taken to choose other diseases not associated with the exposure of interest. Otherwise, the comparison of the proportion exposed among the cases and controls will not be valid, in that the exposure proportion among the controls will not be a valid reflection of the proportion to be expected among all those who are hospitalized without the disease of interest. For example, as controls for lung cancer cases in a study of lung cancer and smoking it would not be good to choose as controls those with other nonmalignant respiratory disease (e.g., emphysema, bronchitis), since these diseases are associated with smoking.

Even when such care is taken in choosing controls, in hospital case-control studies the results are applicable only to the underlying population that uses the hospital or hospitals.

Case-control studies nested within cohorts are done after the cohort has been followed and cases of the disease of interest identified. At that point, the cases and a random selection of noncases may be evaluated for detailed exposure histories that might have been too expensive to evaluate for the entire cohort originally. Nested case-control studies often are done in an occupational setting. After follow-up and selection of cases and controls, the investigator can examine work history and exposure levels in given jobs in detail. He or she may also choose to contact cases and controls (or their next of kin) for interviews to determine other risk factors, such as smoking history and diet. When there are no nonexposed individuals in the cohort, nested case-control studies often assess the degree of exposure (e.g., high versus low) of cases versus controls. The results of case-control studies nested within cohorts are applicable only to the cohort itself.

A type of study that does not fit clearly into the category of a case-control study is the proportionate mortality study. In a proportionate mortality study, the investigator has as his or her observations the decedents in a hypothetical exposed cohort (for example, deaths among members of a union of granite cutters), compared to the decedents in a nonexposed cohort (e.g., the U.S. population). No information is available on survivors among the exposed group. Hence the exposed cohort as a whole is not identified. Among the deaths, the investigator hypothesizes that the proportion resulting from a specific cause (e.g., lung cancer) will be higher than expected if the exposure of interest (e.g., granite dust) increases the risk of that cause of death. The proportion of deaths due to a specific cause among the exposed is compared to the proportion in the nonexposed group (e.g., the U.S. population), to form a proportionate mortality ratio. If this ratio is greater than one, then the investigator may conclude that the exposure is associated with the cause of death.

Proportionate mortality studies suffer from the well-known problem that the proportions of deaths from different causes are not independent; a deficit in one cause will lead to an excess of another cause. For example, workers often die less of heart disease than the general population (the "healthy worker effect"). Hence, the proportion of deaths from heart disease may be low in a working population compared to the U.S. population. This will tend to artificially increase the proportion of cancer deaths in the exposed group, and might lead the investigator to falsely conclude that exposure is associated with cancer.

Proportionate mortality studies are easier to carry out than full cohort studies, and frequently give similar answers. The proportionate mortality ratio (PMR) for a given cause in an exposed versus a nonexposed population is often similar to the rate ratio (e.g., the SMR) for that cause, which would have been obtained if a full cohort study had been conducted. This will be true if the SMR for all causes between exposed and nonexposed is approximately 1.00 (although typically this cannot be known when a PMR analysis is under consideration).

An alternative analysis to a proportionate mortality analysis is a case-control analysis of the same decedents (Miettenin and Wang, 1981). This is especially useful when there is a group of nonexposed or low-exposed among the decedents, so an internal analysis can be done instead of using as the referent group an external population. A case-control analysis can avoid the problems of competing causes mentioned above, by excluding control deaths known to be linked to exposure (internal analyses also avoid the healthy worker effect).

Consider the data below.

	Case-Control		Proportionate Mortality	
	Case (lung cancer)	Control (other deaths)	Lung Cancer Deaths	Total Deaths
Exp	a	b	a	a + b
Non-exp	c	d	c	c + d
	Ratio of odds = ad/bc		Ratio of proportions = $\frac{a/a + b}{c/b + d}$	

The odds ratio resulting from a case-control analysis and the proportionate mortality ratio (internal analyses) will be approximately equal if the cause of death of interest is rare (so that a/a + b is approximately equal to a/b).

In Part II there are three chapters devoted to case-control studies and one to a proportionate mortality study. The first case-control study is a population-based study of end-stage renal disease in Michigan, in which matched controls are chosen via random-digit dialing. The second case-control study is nested within a traditional cohort mortality study of vinyl chloride workers. The third case-control study is restricted to decedents and is nested within a cohort of pensioners in the Teamsters Union. The proportionate mortality study is a study of lung cancer among granite cutters, in which the U.S. population is used as the nonexposed population.

References

Miettinen O, Wang J: An alternative to the proportionate mortality ratio. Am J Epidemiol 114,1:144–148, 1991.

Chapter 4 | A Case-Control Study of End-Stage Renal Disease

KYLE STEENLAND

Numerous case reports have indicated that acute renal failure can follow high exposures to metals, solvents, and silica. In addition, several case-control studies have indicated an association between chronic renal disease (particularly glomerulonephritis) and long-term solvent exposure. Several follow-up studies have also suggested that long-term exposure to lead and uranium may lead to chronic renal disease. While these reports and epidemiologic studies have been suggestive, the role of occupational exposures to metals, solvents, and silica in causing nonmalignant renal disease is by no means clear.

Nonmalignant renal disease can lead to renal failure, or end-stage renal disease (ESRD). ESRD is a serious condition, with a five-year survival rate of less than 50%. The incidence rate for ESRD is approximately 6 per 100,000. There are over 120,000 Americans who have end-stage renal disease (ESRD). Without functioning kidneys, these patients must receive a kidney transplant or be maintained on dialysis. There are approximately 40,000 new cases of ESRD per year, and treatment costs exceed $2 billion annually. Despite this enormous public health burden, little is known about the causes of most renal disease.

The current study was designed to test the hypothesis that occupational exposures to metals, solvents, and silica are associated with ESRD.

QUESTION 1. What types of study design could be used to study ESRD? Discuss advantages and disadvantages of feasible approaches.

Methods

Investigators decided on a case-control approach, and chose to study ESRD patients (rather than those with less severe renal disease). Cases were available from a state registry of ESRD patients in Michigan. Cases were restricted to males who had been diagnosed with ESRD between 1976 and 1984 and who were age 30 to 69 at diagnosis. Cases also had to have been alive in 1984 when the study was begun. ESRD patients who had been diagnosed with congenital, obstructive, diabetic, or heroin nephropathy were excluded from the case series, as were a small number of patients with renal syndromes with a important genetic component. The cases who were included generally had ESRD subsequent to glomerulonephritis, nephrosclerosis, and interstitial disease. These diagnoses represented about 65% of the ESRD patients in Michigan. Finally, cases were restricted to three urban areas of Michigan (Detroit, Flint/Saginaw, and Lansing). Controls were to be chosen via random-digit dialing from the general population, and pair-matched to the cases by sex, age, race, and geographic area. Both cases and controls would be interviewed by telephone to determine work history and other nonoccupational exposures.

QUESTION 2. What different kinds of case-control studies could be conducted? Why did investigators choose to use a statewide registry as their source of cases?

QUESTION 3a. Why were cases restricted to ESRD subsequent to particular types of renal disease?

QUESTION 3b. Why were they restricted by sex and geographical area?

QUESTION 3c. Why were they restricted by age?

QUESTION 3d. Why were they required to be alive in 1984?

QUESTION 4. Why were controls to be pair-matched to cases on age, race, sex, and geographical area?

The Michigan Kidney Registry identified 612 eligible cases who had been diagnosed as end-stage from 1976 to 1984, but who were known to still be alive in 1984. Investigators chose this range of years so that they would be able to select approximately 600 cases. This number was desired because it was felt that if the response rate was at least 50%, then at least 300 cases would be available, and power calculations indicated that with 300 cases, reasonably small relative risks for occupational exposures could be detected. Budgetary constraints precluded contacting and interviewing more than a total sample size (cases and controls) of approximately 600 to 700 people.

QUESTION 5. Assume that the investigators required 80% power (Z_{beta} of 0.84), and a rejection or alpha level of 5% (Z_{alpha} of 1.96). Assume also that 10% of the controls are exposed (P_0), compared to 18% of the cases (P_1) (yielding an odds ratio of about 2.00). Assume equal numbers of cases and controls will be used and then use the formula in the Appendix to determine the number of cases and controls required to attain the specified 80% power. This formula applies to unmatched studies, but can be used as a reasonable approximation for a matched study such as this one. Suppose 20% of the controls are exposed, versus 30% of the cases (an odds ratio of about 1.7). How many cases and controls will then be required?

Controls were chosen via random-digit dialing, and were pair-matched to cases by age (within five years), and geographical area defined by three-digit telephone prefixes (the first three numbers of the seven-digit telephone number). There were 15 different geographical areas. Random-digit dialing was conducted within each geographical area by generating random phone numbers. These numbers were then called until a household was found with a control willing to participate and matching the age and race of some case in that geographical area.

Both cases and controls were interviewed by phone regarding work history and nonoccupational variables. Interviews took approximately 30 minutes, and were conducted by trained interviewers using a standard text. It was impossible to blind interviewers to case-control status because the case's illness was often apparent upon interview, and because cases frequently referred to their disease in answering specific questions.

Questions were asked regarding prolonged and regular use of pain pills prior to renal disease (more than one pill per week for two years or more), prolonged and regular drinking of moonshine whiskey, education, smoking, and family history of kidney disease (for first-degree relatives only). Family history of renal disease excluded kidney stones and kidney cancer, or renal disease known to have occurred subsequent to diabetes or trauma. Responses for pain pills were classified according to whether the pain pill included phenacetin or acetaminophen.

Occupational questions were asked regarding all jobs held for more than six months past the age of 18. For each job, subjects reported occupation and industry, and were asked about regular (not occasional) exposure to solvents, silica, metal fumes, metal particles, oil/gas, mercury, and ammonia. Questions regarding these specific exposures included brief examples of processes in which these exposures typically occur. For positive responses, the process in which the exposure occurred was recorded, as well as the approximate hours per week of exposure. Industrial hygienists reviewed the reported exposures after the interview. When necessary, subjects were reinterviewed to clarify questions about any exposures that appeared inconsistent or implausible.

Occupational and nonoccupational exposures were truncated for both cases and controls at the year at which the index case was diagnosed with ESRD.

QUESTION 6. Interviews are conducted "blindly," whenever possible, so that the interviewer does not know whether the subject is a case or control. That was impossible in this study. What biases could have been introduced by this lack of "blindness."

With the exception of smoking and ammonia, the exposures asked about in the questionnaire were suspected of being associated with kidney disease. Questions about smoking habits were asked because smoking is associated with many diseases and questions on smoking are frequently included even when no prior association has been established. The question on ammonia was included as a check on "recall bias."

QUESTION 7. Can you explain what "recall bias" is and how the ammonia question might help uncover it?

Results

Full results for this study may be found in Steenland et al. (1990).

Of the 612 eligible cases, 87 died prior to any attempt to contact them, and 14 died after consenting to be interviewed but prior to the interview's taking place. Another 26 were found to be ineligible because upon interview their renal disease was found to be subsequent to diabetes or heroin abuse, which were ineligible diagnostic categories. Fourteen others could not participate because they were in jail or mentally incompetent. Of the remaining 471 men, investigators interviewed 325 (69%).

For controls, 3,962 numbers were called, with an average of two calls per number. Of these, 61% were working residential numbers. Of these, in turn, 23% refused to provide initial information regarding household males. For those households who did provide information and did have eligible males, investigators interviewed 79%.

QUESTION 8. From the above two paragraphs, comment on the oft-made assertion that case-control studies are generally less expensive and time-consuming than cohort studies.

QUESTION 9. In this study, how would you calculate a response rate for cases and controls? Do you think the response rate is sufficiently high among cases?

Table 4.1 provides selected variables for cases and controls, without taking the pair-matching into account.

QUESTION 10. Why are the number of nonwhites the same in each group, and why are the average years of birth so similar?

QUESTION 11. Most risk factors in Table 4.1 appear to be somewhat or

TABLE 4.1 Results for Selected Variables by Case-Control Status

Variable	Cases (n = 325)	Controls (n = 325)
Average years of education	11.7	12.5
Some college	106	129
Number of nonwhites	143	143
Average date of birth	1930	1931
Family kidney disease	37	7
Regular moonshine use	31	10
Regular use of phenacetin/acetaminophen	22	7
Current cigarette smokers	143	151
Former cigarette smokers	119	91
Ever regularly exposed, solvents	124	82
Ever regularly exposed, metal fumes	139	94
Ever regularly exposed, metal particles	119	96
Ever regularly exposed, oil/gas	135	129
Ever regularly exposed, silica	87	54
Ever regularly exposed, ammonia	33	19

strongly associated with ESRD, including ammonia. Do you think this is due to recall bias on the part of the cases? Can you think of an alternative explanation?

QUESTION 12. Can you think of a reason that current (at time of ESRD diagnosis) smokers are *less* common among cases?

QUESTION 13. For solvent exposure, there were 25 pairs of cases and controls in which both case and controls were exposed. There were 99 pairs in which only the case was exposed, and 57 in which only the control was exposed.

Calculate the crude (or unadjusted) odds ratio for solvent exposure using the method appropriate for matched-pair data, as well as the odds ratio without regard to matching. Calculate the McNemar chi-square test of association for solvent exposure appropriate for matched-pair data, and calculate the usual Mantel-Haenszel chi-square statistic without regard for matching. Compare the results for the odds ratio and the test of association with and without taking matching into account. Comment on whether it makes much difference whether matching is ignored in this analysis.

QUESTION 14. What is lacking in the analysis for solvent exposure in Question 13? What further analyses must be conducted? Can you think of any limitations in using stratified analysis to conduct these further analyses?

Table 4.2 presents results from the multivariate analyses for the primary variables of interest. The multivariate model included a core group of nonoccupational variables, which were year of birth (continuous), family history (0/1), moonshine use (0/1), and years of schooling (continuous).

The odds ratios, for a number of variables, are lower than the crude or unadjusted univariate ones. For example, the crude odds ratios (matching retained) for phenacetin/acetaminophen, moonshine, solvents, and silica were 3.14, 3.33, 1.74, and 1.89, respectively, all statistically significant. The lower adjusted odds ratios reflect control of positive confounding by other variables, such as years of education, as well as mutual confounding among several of the variables listed above. The multivariate analyses was able to dissipate some of the concerns about recall bias discussed in Question and Answer 11. Note that while the odds ratio for ammonia is still elevated, it is no longer statistically significant.

QUESTION 15. Do the odds ratios by subcategory of solvent, silica, and metal fume exposure strengthen the argument that these exposures are

TABLE 4.2 Results from Multivariate Analyses

Variable	Odds Ratio (95% CI)
Phenacetin/acetaminophen	2.66 (1.04–6.82)
Family history	9.30 (7.99–10.82)
Moonshine	2.42 (1.10–5.36)
Solvents (all)	1.51 (1.03–2.22)
Used in paints/glues	1.10 (0.58–1.74)
Used as degreasers	2.50 (1.56–3.95)
Used elsewhere	1.05 (0.44–1.28)
Metal fumes (all)	1.17 (0.77–1.80)
Lead (mostly soldering)	1.73 (0.82–3.65)
Welding	0.75 (0.44–1.28)
Metal particles	0.97 (0.58–1.48)
Oil and gas	0.74 (0.64–1.51)
Silica (all)	1.67 (1.02–2.74)
Cement and sand	0.78 (0.34–1.78)
Brick and foundry	1.92 (1.06–3.46)
Sandblasting	3.83 (0.97–15.19)
Used elsewhere	1.08 (0.42–2.77)
Ammonia	1.31 (0.66–2.60)

truly associated with ESRD? What further analyses could be done to test these associations?

Further analyses were conducted for phenacetin/acetaminophen and moonshine use by frequency and duration of exposure. Similarly, for occupational variables, analyses were conducted by duration of exposure. These variables were used as surrogates for cumulative dose, for which data were lacking. For the occupational variables, duration of exposure was calculated by multiplying the hours per week exposed by the years in a given job, and summing this product over all jobs, for each exposure of interest. Results for these analyses showed increasing trends for duration and frequency of phenacetin/acetaminophen and moonshine exposure, although these trends fell short of statistical significance. For the occupational variables, generally there was little or no evidence of increasing risk with increasing duration of exposure, although the trend for sandblasting was highly positive and approached statistical significance.

Yet another analysis used a job-exposure matrix to analyze for increasing risk with increasing likelihood and intensity of solvent exposure. This matrix was created by industrial hygienists, independently of the study discussed here. The job exposure assigned a probability-of-exposure score and an intensity-of-exposure score to all occupations (by industry) with any probability of solvent exposure. The product of the probability score and the intensity score was used as an overall measure of solvent exposure.

QUESTION 16. How exactly was the trend (if any) of increasing risk with increasing duration of exposure (say, to solvents) assessed in the analysis? How was the statistical significance of any observed trends assessed? What are the limitations of an analysis using cumulative duration instead of cumulative dose? What are the limitations of using the job-exposure matrix approach?

QUESTION 17. (optional) Course instructors may obtain a condensed data set on diskette from the author. Table 4.3 shows the data format. Use conditional logistic regression to confirm the results presented above. Why is YRBTH a significant predictor in the model, given that it was a matching variable? Test the variable "RACE" in the model. Interpret the result. Interpret the result for the continuous variable "SCHL." Can you find any interaction terms that contribute significantly to the model? Given the relatively high coefficient for "HRSAN," explain why its confidence interval is so wide.

Discussion

This population-based case-control study discovered some significant associations between both occupational and nonoccupational exposure and ESRD.

TABLE 4.3 Variables in ESRD Data Set (n = 650)

CASE	YRBTH	RACE	SCHL	YRSPHE	MOON	XWKMN	FAM
1	23	1	23	0	0	0	0
1	27	0	11	0	0	0	0

CASE	FAM2	SOL	MET	SIL	PHE	HRSOL	HRSAN	ID
1	1	1	1	0	0	111	0	1
CASE	1	1	0	0	0	128	0	2
1								
. . .								

CASE: 1 = case, 0 = control; YRBRTH: year of birth; RACE: 1 = white, 0 = nonwhite; SCHL: yeas of school; YRSPHE: years of regular use of phenacetin/acetaminophen; MOON: ever regular use of moonshine; XWKMN: times/week use of moonshine when using; FAM: family history of renal disease, excluding stones, cancer, trauma, or renal diseae subsequent to diabetes (1 = yes, 0 = no), first-degree relatives only; FAM2: did not know family history (1 = didn't know, 0 = knew); SOL: ever regular exposure to solvents at work; MET: ever regular exposure to metal fumes at work; SIL: ever regular exposure to silica at work; PHE: ever regular use of phenacetin/acetaminophen; HRSOL: total hours of solvent exposure at work; HRSAN: total hours sandblasting; ID: matching variable to match cases and corresponding controls (1–325).

Suspected associations between moonshine whisky and phenacetin/acetamino-phen use were confirmed, and upward but not significant trends with increasing duration and frequency of exposure were noted for these variables. A strong relationship was found with family history, which was an unsuspected new finding. This finding could be partly an artifact, because hypertension is familial and hypertension causes renal disease. Suspected associations with solvents and silica were also confirmed. A positive but nonsignificant finding (also suspected a priori) was noted for lead. Furthermore, the subcategories of solvent and silica exposure that showed the most risk for ESRD were the ones most likely to have involved higher exposures.

On the other hand, for the occupational variables there were no trends of increased risk with increased duration of exposure, which somewhat weakens the case for true occupational associations.

One of the weaknesses of the study was that it was not possible to conduct separate analyses by type of renal disease leading to ESRD. This was so because it was felt that the diagnoses in the Registry were not sufficiently accurate to differentiate between the categories of hypertensive, glomerular, and interstitial disease. This was one of the disadvantages of studying ESRD patients: many patients come to diagnosis without prior treatment and most lack any biopsy data, making a definitive diagnosis difficult.

References

Steenland K, Thun M, Ferguson, W, et al.: Occupational and other exposures associated with male end-stage renal disease: a case-control study. Am J Pub Health 80,2:153–157, 1990.

ANSWERS

ANSWER 1. A cross-sectional approach is not possible for a chronic disease that is a rare and debilitating condition. A cohort approach would be difficult because there are a variety of exposures of interest, and it would be difficult to assemble a cohort with all these exposures represented. Furthermore, the incidence rate for ESRD is not high, and very large cohorts would have to be studied to observe many cases. Such sample-size problems would occur even if the cohorts were studied retrospectively. Determination of who got ESRD in a cohort would be difficult and very expensive, requiring personal contact with each study subject or their next of kin, and the obtaining of medical records. Interviews would be required with each study subject to control for other known factors influencing renal disease (e.g., phenacetin in pain pills, lead in moonshine whiskey). The case-control approach is the most feasible. A large case series could be assembled, interviews could be conducted, and a variety of exposures could be studied simultaneously, including nonoccupational ones. The disadvantage of the case-control approach is that past exposures would be reported by the study subjects themselves, who might have selective or faulty recall.

ANSWER 2. A case series could be assembled from a hospital or several hospitals. A hospital-based study offered several advantages. A hospital-based series would permit the study of all patients with renal disease, whether they went on to end-stage or not. Good medical records characterizing each patient would be available, permitting the choice of only certain types of kidney disease should investigators so desire. A specific cutoff point for "serious" kidney disease could be defined based on objective measures of renal function in the medical record.

On the other hand, hospital-based case-control series sometimes suffer from several problems. Results are not applicable to the general population but only to the segments of the population that use the hospital(s). The population that uses the hospital may be exposed to the agent of interest more or less than the general population. Logistically, to assemble a large number of patients with serious renal disease might well require working with several hospitals, and obtaining physician clearances to contact patients might prove a major task.

The alternative actually chosen was to assemble a "population-based" case series of ESRD patients from a statewide registry. The cost of treatment of ESRD (dialysis may cost as much as $30,000 a year) is usually paid by the federal government, and regional lists of ESRD patients are maintained by federal authorities. These lists have facilitated the development of statewide registries, which are known to include virtually all ESRD patients in the state. A complete registry makes possible a population-based case-control study, where all the new cases of ESRD in a given area over a given period of time are studied, and a sample of the nondiseased in that same geographical area (the "base" population) serve as controls. ESRD registries are computerized, and include summary diagnostic data regarding the type of renal disease that resulted in ESRD. The ease of obtaining a case series and the general desirability of a population-based study led to the decision to use a statewide registry as the source of cases. This decision meant restricting the study to end-stage cases.

ANSWER 3a. Some types of renal disease are congenital, others can result from trauma or heroin abuse, and still others are known to have a strong genetic component. Occupational exposures are unlikely to play a role in these types of renal disease, and therefore these types of ESRD cases were excluded. Many ESRD cases result from diabetes. While occupational exposures could increase the risk of diabetic nephropathy, diabetics have a high risk of ESRD absent any other exposures, and investigators also excluded diabetic cases. These exclusions were based on the summary diagnosis in the Registry. Complete medical records were not available from Registry data, however, and the diagnosis in the Registry may not always have been accurate.

ANSWER 3b. While there was no theoretical reason to limit cases to a particular sex or geographical area, there was a practical one. The occupational exposures of interest in this study were more common among males and city residents than among females and rural residents. The sample size required to detect a given level of effect increases when the prevalence of the exposure among the nondiseased is quite small. Budget constraints required that the proposed study be limited to a certain sample size, so it was desirable that the prevalence of exposure among the controls be as high as possible. Therefore, investigators decided to restrict the study to males living in urban areas.

ANSWER 3c. There are very few ESRD patients under age 30. Patients aged 70+ were excluded because they are also fewer in number, and because they might not be living at home and therefore easily interviewable by phone.

ANSWER 3d. Cases were required to be alive in 1984 (at the time of data collection) because it was felt that a reliable work history, going back in time and sufficiently detailed to identify specific exposures, could not be obtained from surrogate respondents such as next of kin.

ANSWER 4. Matching in a case-control study is often done to control for confounding, which might result from the matching variables if no matching were used. However, use of a matched design generally requires maintaining the matching in the analysis. The effects of the matching variables themselves on the disease, then, cannot be estimated in the analysis. Usually one matches on variables known to be strongly related to disease that are not of inherent interest and that might differ between exposed and nonexposed (and therefore be confounders). This is the case here with age, race, and sex, which are all associated with renal disease and could have differed between exposed and nonexposed groups. In Michigan, the relative risk of ESRD for blacks compared to whites is about 4.3, while the relative risk for males compared to females is about 1.4 (Weller et al., 1985). Another reason for matching is to control indirectly the effects of a series of unmeasured variables (such as diet and socioeconomic status) suspected of being confounders, via another surrogate variable like geographical residence. Pair-matching as opposed to frequency matching or R-to-1 matching was used for logistical convenience and to maximize the number of cases studied given the overall limit on sample size due to budgetary constraints.

ANSWER 5. The formula in the Appendix relates power (1-B), the rejection level (alpha), sample size (n_0 is the number of controls needed), exposure prevalence among controls (P_0), and exposure prevalence among cases (P_1) for an unmatched case-control study.

When the exposure prevalence among controls and cases is 10% and 18%, respectively (odds ratio of 1.95), the number of cases (and controls) needed is 289, if an 80% power is to be achieved with a rejection level of 5% (alpha). Similarly, if the prevalences are 20% and 30%, respectively (odds ratio of 1.7), then 292 cases and 292 controls are needed. Investigators in this study, who knew they could afford to obtain about 300 cases and 300 controls, therefore knew they had reasonable power to detect true relative risks on the order of 1.7–2.0, assuming exposure prevalences among controls were about 10 to 20%. Such relative risks were plausible based on the existing literature, and the assumed prevalences also appeared reasonable, so that the study was judged to be worth conducting.

ANSWER 6. The concern is that interviewers may probe more deeply for exposures among the cases, resulting in false positive results due to interviewer bias. This kind of bias is avoided by employing trained interviewers who do not deviate from prepared scripts and questionnaires. Pretests of the script and questionnaire are essential.

ANSWER 7. Recall bias can be a major problem in collecting occupational and other history in case-control studies. Recall bias occurs when cases overreport exposures compared to controls because they take the questions more seriously than controls and make a greater effort to answer them. Overreporting by cases can also occur because cases are eager to attribute their illness to virtually any identifiable past exposures. If recall bias is at work, cases would be expected to overreport all exposures, not just those suspected of causing renal disease (assuming the cases do not know which exposures are suspected a priori). In this study, investigators therefore included one question on a substance thought *not* to be related to renal disease (ammonia). If cases over-reported all exposures, then resulting odds ratios would be high for all exposures, including ammonia, indicating that positive results may have been due to recall bias.

ANSWER 8. While case-control studies usually involve far fewer subjects than cohort studies, they can involve much higher costs per subject. Interview studies always involve a higher cost per subject than record-based studies. Occupational cohort mortality studies are often done with records alone, without contacting the subject. Case-control studies, which by their nature often involve direct interview with study subjects to ascertain past exposures, can be very expensive due to interview costs (e.g., $100 per interview). If random-digit dialing is used to obtain controls, costs increase further (e.g., $100 per control obtained).

ANSWER 9. There are many ways of calculating a response rate. In this study investigators calculated a response rate of 69% for interviewing eligible cases and 79% for interviewing eligible controls. Among eligible cases, nonrespondents were more likely than respondents to be nonwhite (67% versus 44%) and live in the inner city of Detroit (61% versus 40%). Controls showed a similar pattern. If the nonrespondents differed sub-stantially in their exposures, then the interviewed group may not have been representative of the eligible population and estimates of exposure effect may have been biased.

Another issue is that the "eligible" population of cases represented the survivors of those diagnosed with ESRD during the 1976–1984 study period. Another 484 men who would have been eligible had died. These men differed little from the eligible group with respect to race or resi-dence, but were approximately five years older. Had their exposures been substantially different from those studied (there is no good a priori reason to suspect this), the studied cases might have been unrepresen-tative.

ANSWER 10. Controls were matched to cases on race and date of birth (within five years).

ANSWER 11. There are several explanations possible. One explanation is recall bias: the cases remember past exposures better (or more) than controls. A second possibility is that most of these exposures are indeed causally related to ESRD, although this seems a priori unlikely. A third possibility is that cases are more likely to have held blue-collar jobs than controls, and hence indeed were more commonly exposed to all the occupational agents considered. There is support for this last possibility in the data on education, in that cases were less likely to have been to college. As a result, they may have been more likely to have had more blue-collar jobs and more workplace exposures than controls. It is not clear *why* cases had less education than controls. It could be that controls with more education were more likely to participate in random-digit dialing than controls with less education, in contrast to cases, although the literature on random-digit dialing does not suggest this. It could be that other, unknown, factors associated with poverty may increase the risk of ESRD, although again this is not indicated in the literature.

ANSWER 12. Most patients were ill prior to diagnosis of ESRD, and may have quit smoking during their illness. Note that former smokers are more prevalent among cases. However, considering current and former smokers together, there are still more ever-smokers among cases than among controls. Given that fewer cases than controls went to college, smoking differences may reflect the well-known phenomenon that college-educated populations tend to have lower smoking rates. Although smoking was associated with disease in this study, it did not act as a confounder for the occupational variables of interest and was not included in final models. This implies that smoking was not associated with exposure.

ANSWER 13. The odds ratio for matched-pair data is the ratio of discordant pairs, which is 99/57, or 1.74. The usual odds ratio for unmatched data, based on a single table, is 1.83, slightly higher. The McNemar test of association, which is equivalent to a Mantel-Haenszel test over 325 strata in which each strata is composed of a matched pair, is $(99-57)^2 / 156$, or 11.3, which is highly significant. The usual chi-square for a single 2×2 table is 12.5, somewhat higher (not surprising, given that the odds ratio is also slightly higher). These results are quite comparable, but the correct results are those that take the matching into account (see Answer 14 as well).

ANSWER 14. The crude analysis for solvent exposure failed to correct for confounding by other variables. We have already noted (answer 11) that years of education may be a confounder in these data, and that one occupational variable may confound another. In addition, family history, pain pill use, and moonshine whiskey use were strongly related to ESRD in this study and therefore (if they were also related to occupational exposures) could have been acting as confounders for an analysis of solvent exposure. To control for possible confounding, an analysis with several variables considered simultaneously is necessary. This cannot be done via stratification for pair-matched data. Consider stratification in order to control for education. The investigators would need to stratify all pairs by level of education, considering those with some college educa- tion and those without college education separately, for example. Yet some matched pairs will be discordant for college education, making it impossible to allocate both members of the pair to one strata of educa- tion or the other. Instead, a multivariate analysis must be done via a conditional logistic regression model, which not only enables the simul- taneous consideration of many variables while retaining the pair-match- ing, but also permits the use of continuous variables as well as discrete or dichotomous ones.

ANSWER 15. Yes, they do. The subcategories of silica and solvent exposures that have the highest odds ratios also involve higher ex- posures. Sandblasting is likely to involve the highest silica exposures, followed by foundries, while exposure to sand and cement involves very little exposure to free silica. Similarly, using solvents as degreasers involves higher exposures than being exposed to solvents in paints and glues. Regarding metal fumes, there is an a priori suspicion that lead exposure is associated with renal disease. Further analyses along these lines would test for a trend of increased risk with increased exposure (dose-response). Since actual doses are lacking for this study (as is true in most case-control studies), a surrogate (e.g., duration of exposure) might be used.

ANSWER 16. A variable for cumulative duration of exposure was put in the conditional logistic regression model, and its coefficient estimated. If the coefficient was positive, this indicated an increasing risk of ESRD with increasing duration of exposure. The significance of any trend (positive or negative) was determined by whether the coefficient for the duration variable was statistically significant—that is, significantly different from zero.
   The limitation of using duration as a surrogate for dose is that it may be a poor surrogate, because it ignores level or intensity of exposure. For example, short high exposure will be treated the same as short low exposure, but will result in a higher cumulative dose. The job-exposure matrix approach has its own limitations. An a priori assignment of the

likelihood and intensity of exposure to solvents for all occupations is necessarily a crude measure of exposure. The job-exposure matrix essentially ignores all the self-reported data on exposure available from the interviews, and relies solely on occupational title. This can be an advantage in that it avoids reliance on the subjectivity of the study subject in reporting specific exposures to solvents, but a disadvantage in that it replaces a person's own report of exposure with a hygienist's assessment of whether a job is likely to entail solvent exposure. Attempts to validate job-exposure matrices have not often succeeded (for example, using a job-exposure matrix to predict which people in a population are exposed to asbestos, yet not finding any excess lung cancer risk in people so identified).

ANSWER 17. If each case-control pair has exactly the same value for a variable, no odds ratio is calculable. This is the case for RACE. YRBTH, on the other hand, was matched only within five years. The fact that this variable is a significant predictor with a negative coefficient means that on the average, for each case-control pair, the controls were born later than the cases. SCHL has a negative coefficient, meaning that fewer years of school increases the risk of ESRD. Interaction terms are generally insignificant in the model. Few people were sandblasters, so the coefficient for HRSAN is unstable, with high variance, resulting in a wide confidence interval.

References for Answers

Weller J, Wu S, Ferguson W, et al.: End-stage renal disease in Michigan. Am J Nephrol 5:84–95, 1985.

Chapter 5

A Vinyl Chloride Case-Control Study

KYLE STEENLAND

In 1972, investigators from the National Institute for Occupational Safety and Health (NIOSH) were informed of a report of a cluster of liver cancers at a plant in Louisville, Kentucky, that produced polyvinyl chloride (PVC) plastic products. This plant opened in 1942 and produced both the monomer gas (VC gas) and the polymerized plastic (PVC) through 1966. In 1966, the plant stopped production of VC gas, but continued to buy the gas and to produce PVC products. About three-quarters of the men who had worked at the plant had been exposed to both VC gas and PVC dust.

NIOSH conducted a cohort mortality study of workers exposed to VC gas between 1942 and 1973 at this plant (Waxweiler et al., 1976). NIOSH investigators collected personnel records (demographic data and work history) in late 1973 at the plant, for all employees past and present. However, the analysis of these data was restricted to men with at least five years employment at the plant, and at least ten years since first employment at the plant. In comparison to the nonexposed U.S. population, this study showed statistically significant excesses of lung (12 observed, SMR = 1.56), brain (3 observed, SMR = 3.33), and liver (7 observed, SMR = 11.66) cancers.

While exact levels of exposure to VC gas and PVC dust at the plant were not known, NIOSH investigators did rank different jobs in the plant according to the estimated level of exposure to both VC and PVC dust. These rankings were not used in the initial cohort study, although they were used in subsequent case-control analyses of the cohort (Waxweiler et al., 1981; Smith et al., 1980). Exposures to VC gas decreased markedly after 1974, when the Occupational Safety and Health Administration (OSHA) lowered the standard for exposure to VC gas to 1 part per million (ppm).

Despite many studies of vinyl chloride since 1973, in the late 1980s several questions remained. While it was accepted that VC gas caused liver cancer, it will still unclear whether either VC gas or PVC dust caused other cancers, principally of the lung and brain. PVC dust was of particular concern because relatively large numbers of workers continue to be exposed to PVC dust, while few workers are still exposed to VC gas (and those at very low levels). In 1987, investigators at NIOSH turned back to their original data collected at the Louisville plant in an attempt to answer these questions.

QUESTION 1. What study design or designs could be used to answer these unresolved questions regarding VC gas and PVC dust?

Methods

Investigators chose to conduct a new cohort mortality study of all male workers at the plant (not just those exposed to VC gas). Depending on the results of the new cohort study, case-control studies of lung, brain, and liver cancer, "nested" within the cohort, were tentatively planned to study specific exposures and dose-response.

The new cohort mortality study would have vital status follow-up through 1986. No new exposure information was to be collected, and the cohort was to be restricted to those employed at the plant at any time between 1942 and 1973.

QUESTION 2a. Why did investigators choose to conduct a new cohort mortality study (followed by case-control studies) instead of an incidence study?

QUESTION 2b. What is meant by "vital status follow-up through 1986"? What is the purpose of vital status follow-up?

QUESTION 2c. Why did investigators restrict the cohort to those who worked at the plant between 1942 and 1973?

QUESTION 2d. Why had the original investigators chosen to restrict their analyses to those men exposed to VC gas and those with at least ten years since first employment and at least five years employment?

QUESTION 2e. Could the new vital status follow-up have been restricted to these same men, saving time and money?

Results

Full results for this study, with follow-up through 1986, were published by Wu et al. (1989). Table 5.1 shows the follow-up information through 1986. Note

TABLE 5.1 Vital Status Follow-up

Vital Status	Total Cohort (%)	VC Cohort (%)
Alive	3,620 (75)	2,767 (76)
Dead	1,181 (24)	843 (23)
Unknown	34 (1)	25 (1)
Person/yrs at risk	139,106	103,368

that investigators divided the total cohort into everyone at the plant and those exposed to VC gas.

Table 5.2 shows the results for observed and expected deaths for the VC cohort, in the cohort analysis.

QUESTION 3. Given these results, do you think further case-control studies were warranted for lung, liver, and brain cancer?

Three separate case-control studies were conducted. Cases for these studies consisted of all those workers (men and women) at the plant who had died of the three causes of interest. For each case, five matched controls were chosen.

In case-control studies, the controls are chosen to be a representative sample of the nondiseased population. The exposures of the cases are then compared to the controls. There are a variety of methods of choosing controls. In this study, cases occurred over a long period of time (1942 to 1986), and it was desirable to take time into account in choosing controls, rather than simply choosing controls at random from those who had not died of the cancers of interest. Five matched controls for each case were randomly chosen from all those who were alive at the age when the index case died of the disease. The work history of controls was considered only up to that point in time. For example, if a case died of liver cancer at age 50, five controls were selected randomly from cohort members who were alive at age 50. The work history of the selected controls was considered only up to age 50. This procedure meant that cases and their five controls were matched on age. Controls were also matched to their index case by race and sex.

TABLE 5.2 VC Cohort Results

Causes of Death	Observed	Expected	SMR (95% CI)
All deaths	843	885.7	95 (90–101)
Lung cancer	80	69.2	115 (95–139)
Brain cancer	10	6.8	145 (79–248)
Liver cancer	14	4.2	333 (202–521)

Table 5.3 lists the number of cases and controls for each disease, and the percentage ever exposed to VC gas and PVC dust. Exposure (ever/never) status was determined after a review of the jobs held by each individual, and a knowledge of which jobs had exposure and which did not.

Table 5.3 shows that most study subjects were exposed to VC gas and PVC dust, as expected. Frequently, if a worker was exposed to one agent, he or she was also exposed to the other. This meant that it would not be possible to separate the effects of VC gas and PVC dust when exposure was coded as "ever/never." However, some jobs did involve exposure to gas and not to dust, and vice versa. Furthermore, levels of exposure to gas or dust varied by job. Hence, another measure of exposure that took into account *level* of exposure might allow the separation of the effects of VC gas and PVC dust.

In comparing the exposures of cases to controls in data such as these, in which each control is matched to a particular case, the analysis must take into account the matching (a matched analysis). However, as an approximation, odds ratios may be calculated using the unmatched data in Table 5.3.

QUESTION 4a. Calculate the odds ratio for liver cancer for ever having been exposed to VC gas, using the unmatched data in the table. Calculate the test of significance for this odds ratio, and the 95% test-based confidence intervals.

QUESTION 4b. This odds ratio is rather low, compared to the SMR of 333 found in the cohort study. Why?

QUESTION 4c. What is the next step in the case-control analysis?

The original investigators had ranked jobs by exposure level to VC gas and PVC dust, with rankings going from 0 (nonexposed) to 5 (most highly exposed). These rankings were done for each year during the plant's history, given that processes and exposures changed over time. The work histories of all cases

TABLE 5.3 Number of Subjects in Case-Control Studies

Disease	Exposed to VC (%)	Exposed to PVC (%)	Total
Liver			
Cases	16 (84)	16 (84)	19
Controls	74 (78)	81 (85)	95
Brain			
Cases	13 (87)	13 (87)	15
Controls	63 (84)	62 (83)	75
Lung			
Cases	96 (84)	98 (86)	114
Controls	475 (83)	456 (80)	570

and controls were reviewed and each job was assigned the appropriate ranking. A cumulative exposure was then calculated by multiplying the exposure level of each job by the number of years in that job, and then summing this product across all jobs held by an individual:

$$\text{Cum Exp} = \sum_{\text{over all jobs}} (\text{level})(\text{years in job})$$

Table 5.4 shows the average cumulative exposure to VC gas and PVC dust for the three case-control studies.

QUESTION 5a. Can you think of other ways to have measured exposure, with the data available?

QUESTION 5b. Do the data in Table 5.4 indicate that either VC gas or PVC dust increases the risk or either liver, brain, or lung cancer?

While the data in Table 5.4 provide a crude indication of important differences in cumulative exposure between cases and controls, the final analysis used a conditional logistic regression model in which cumulative exposure (a quantitative variable) was used to predict which person in each matched set (one case, five controls) was the case. In this model it is possible to include more than one predictor variable (independent variable). For example, the model might include cumulative exposure to VC gas and year of first exposure.

While cumulative exposure to VC gas and PVC dust remained highly correlated ($r = 0.74$), making it difficult to put them both in the model at the same time, each could be tested separately to determine which was a better predictor of disease. Results from such analyses determined that only the association between cumulative exposure to VC gas and liver cancer was statistically significant ($p = .03$). Using the results of the model, the odds ratio for workers

TABLE 5.4 Exposure Levels in Case-Control Studies

Disease	Mean Cumulative Exposure to VC	Mean Cumulative Exposure to PVC
Liver		
Cases	42.8	16.2
Controls	9.6	9.7
Brain		
Cases	14.2	19.0
Controls	14.0	13.5
Lung		
Cases	10.8	10.0
Controls	12.2	11.5

TABLE 5.5 Exposure Levels by Type of Liver Cancer

Disease	Average Cumulative Exposure to VC
Angiosarcoma	61.1
Other liver cancer	11.5
Controls	9.6

exposed at the highest level (level 5) for five years was 7.96 (95% CI 2.17–29.2), compared to those with no exposure.

A further question regarding liver cancer was whether exposure to VC gas was associated just with angiosarcoma of the liver or with other types of liver cancer. Medical records were obtained for the 19 cases of liver cancer, and they were separated between angiosarcoma (n = 12) and other types of liver cancer (n = 7). Cumulative exposures to VC gas were then calculated (Table 5.5) for each type of liver cancer.

QUESTION 6a. How do you interpret the data in Table 5.5?

QUESTION 6b. What are the implications for public health of the overall findings of this study?

Discussion

This study showed that the workers exposed to vinyl chloride gas experienced a significant excess of liver cancer, particularly the rare angiosarcoma of the liver. This excess was related to cumulative dose of vinyl chloride gas. Other cancers suspected a priori (lung and brain) were not found to be associated with exposure to vinyl chloride gas. Exposure to PVC dust was not found to be related to either liver, lung, or brain cancer. These findings for the U.S. cohort were subsequently confirmed by the results of a large multicentric European study of vinyl chloride workers (Simonato et al., 1991).

References

Simonato L, Abbe K, Andersen A, et al.: A collaborative study of cancer incidence and mortality among vinyl chloride workers. Scand J Work Environ Health 17:159–169, 1991.

Smith A, Waxweiler R, Tyroler H: Epidemiologic investigation of occupational carcinogenesis using a serially additive expected dose model. Am J Epidemiol 112,6:787–797, 1980.

Waxweiler R, Smith A, Falk H, et al.: Excess lung cancer risk in a synthetic chemicals plant. Environ Health Perspect 41:159–165, 1981.

Waxweiler R, Stringer W, Wagoner J et al.: Neoplastic risk among workers exposed to vinyl chloride and its polymers. Ann NY Acad Sci 271:40–48, 1976.

Wu W, Steenland K, Brown D, et al.: Cohort and case-control analyses of workers exposed to vinyl chloride: an update. J Occup Med 31,6:518–523, 1989.

ANSWERS

ANSWER 1. Another cohort study of those exposed to VC gas would provide many additional observed deaths, and therefore additional power, to determine whether an excess of liver, brain, or lung continued to exist among these workers. However, it would not answer the questions regarding whether the causal agent was either VC gas or PVC dust. To do this, an analysis was required in which the effects of each of these two agents could be separated. Furthermore, investigators needed to determine whether a dose-response relationship (more exposure leading to more disease) existed between each of these agents (VC gas and PVC dust) and each of the outcomes of concern (liver, lung, and brain cancer). A positive dose-response is one important criterion in determining whether an observed association is causal (see Chapter 2 for a fuller discussion of this issue). In order to investigate a dose-response, investigators would have to use the rankings of each job at the plant by level of exposure to VC gas and PVC dust. The investigators would have to determine whether those men with higher exposures (to either VC gas or PVC dust) were more likely to get cancer.

A nested case-control study could follow a cohort study. In a cohort study in this case, vital status follow-up would be conducted for all current and former plant employees, not jut those exposed to VC gas or PVC dust. Then those who had died of lung cancer, liver cancer, or brain cancer would be identified. A set of nondiseased controls would be selected for each of these three series of cases, and three case-control studies would be conducted. In the case-control studies, the work histories of cases and controls would be compared with respect to level of exposure to VC gas and to PVC dust. One important advantage of the nested case-control study is that detailed exposure histories need only be developed for cases and controls, rather than the entire cohort. Coding and computerizing thousands of detailed work histories is often very time-consuming and expensive.

ANSWER 2a. While disease incidence data is preferable to mortality data (more sensitive), there was no way to determine the cancer incidence of workers at this plant without attempting to contact each cohort member or their next of kin, and then obtaining medical documentation (the United States has no central registry of cancer incidence). This would have been prohibitively expensive.

ANSWER 2b. "Vital status follow-up through 1986" means that the investigators would follow all cohort members through the end of 1986 to determine whether they were alive or dead. For those who died, investigators would obtain their death certificates and determine their cause of death. The analysis based on this follow-up would be that typical of cohort mortality studies. The death rates (observed deaths/person-years at risk) for specific causes in the cohort are compared to the corresponding rates in some nonexposed population (here that of the United States).

ANSWER 2c. Restriction of the cohort to those who worked from 1942 to 1973 meant the investigators did not have to return to the plant to review personnel records, and could restrict their follow-up to those for whom they already had work history. Since exposure was minimal after 1973, the mortality of workers hired after that data was of less interest.

ANSWER 2d. The original investigators restricted their analyses to men exposed to VC gas with at least five years employment and ten years since first employment, because (1) there were very few women (fewer than 5% of the cohort), (2) they were not interested in the mortality of those not exposed to VC gas, and (3) they wanted to consider only those with longer exposures and enough potential latency for a cancer of interest to occur.

ANSWER 2e. In the new follow-up it was necessary to follow all employees, including nonexposed ones, for the purpose of the later case-control studies. In these studies, investigators were planning to assess a dose-response relationship, and here it is important to include those with no exposure and low exposure, so that a range of exposure exists among both cases and controls. Recall that the analysis in the case-control study compares the exposure history of the cases to the controls, seeking to determine if the cases had more exposure. If everyone in the cohort has approximately the same exposures, it is difficult to detect a difference in exposures between cases and controls chosen from within the cohort.

ANSWER 3. All three causes of a priori interest are elevated, although for lung and brain cancer the range of plausible values of the SMR does include 1.0 (no excess). Further work is warranted to determine whether a dose-response relationship exists between either VC gas or PVC dust and any of these three cancers.

ANSWER 4a. The odds ratio of liver cancer for ever having been exposed to VC gas is $(21)(16)/(3)(74)$, or 1.51. The χ^2 statistic is 0.38 (p = .54). Test-based confidence intervals based on this χ^2 are 0.40–5.60 (representing a range of plausible values). Note that the χ^2 calculation is questionable here because of the small number of expecteds in one cell.

ANSWER 4b. The cohort study compared those exposed to VC to the general U.S. population, whereas here the comparison (nonexposed) population are other workers in the same plants. Different comparison populations give different results. Furthermore, the numbers of cases (particularly nonexposed cases) is quite small here, so that the odds ratio is rather unstable or imprecise, which is why the confidence interval is large. Note that the confidence interval includes the result of 3.33 obtained in the cohort study.

ANSWER 4c. The next step is to conduct a dose-response analysis, evaluating whether the level of exposure increases with disease, rather than considering exposure as "ever" versus "never" exposed.

ANSWER 5a. Other ways to measure exposure, which could have been used here, are (1) simple duration of exposure without regard to level, (2) the highest exposure level without regard to duration (peak), and (3) average level of exposure (cumulative exposure divided by duration). A simple measure of duration is generally less preferable to using a cumulative exposure, a combination of level and duration. While peak and average exposure are less common measures of exposure, it is theoretically possible that these measures will be better predictors of disease than either duration or cumulative exposure.

   In general, the best measure of exposure would be actual personal measurements for each person in the study across time. Such exposure data are rarely available, even in the occupational studies where the exposure data are generally better than in environmental studies. One example where such data are available would be workers exposed to radiation who have had badges to measure exposure for many years. Often, however, the best data available to investigators are current sampling measurements for each job in the study, as well as some idea of how the process has changed over time. In this case investigators did not have actual sampling data, but a ranking of jobs within the plant by exposure level, over time. Such a ranking enabled investigators to compare the risk of highly exposed workers to workers with little or no (cumulative) exposure, but did not allow a quantitative assessment of risk per cumulative units of exposure (for example, risk per cumulative parts per million or milligrams/cubic meter air).

ANSWER 5b. The data in Table 5.4 indicate that liver cancer cases have increased exposure to VC gas and PVC dust, compared to controls. There is little indication of differences between cases and controls for the other two cancers.

ANSWER 6a. The data in Table 5.5 indicate that VC gas was only associated with angiosarcoma of the liver.

ANSWER 6b. The fear that PVC dust (a much more common exposure in the general population) was associated with cancer proved unfounded. Furthermore, the fear that VC gas might be a systemic carcinogen, causing many types of cancer including common ones such as lung cancer, also proved unfounded.

Chapter 6

A Case-Control Study of Lung Cancer within the Teamsters Union

KYLE STEENLAND

In the mid-1980s several rodent studies showed that inhaled diesel exhaust caused lung tumors when the exposure levels were relatively high (5–10 mg/cubic meter of diesel particulate) and the exposure period was sufficiently long (NIOSH, 1988). In addition, two studies of railroad workers exposed to diesel fumes suggested an excess lung cancer risk (Howe et al., 1983; Schenker et al., 1984). Given this background, in the mid-1980s investigators at NIOSH decided to study lung cancer risk in another population exposed to diesel exhaust.

QUESTION 1. Without any research, what is your best guess about which workers are exposed to diesel exhaust? Of these, what would be the best population for an epidemiologic study?

Materials and Methods

It was decided to study men exposed to diesel exhaust in the trucking industry. Numerous studies have shown that truck drivers have an excess risk of lung cancer (approximately 50%) (NIOSH, 1988; Hayes et al., 1989). However, a number of these studies have not "controlled" for the effect of smoking, and it is known that truck drivers smoke more than the general population does. Furthermore, none of the existing studies had any information on the levels of exposure to diesel fumes among truck drivers.

It was decided to conduct a study among the members of the Teamsters Union, which is the largest union in the United States. The union had a complete list of all men who had ever qualified for pensions (requiring 20 or more years in the union). For each pensioner, the union had a work history for all union jobs, with employer, occupation, and dates. If a pensioner died, the union obtained the death certificate. Often the union continued paying benefits to the survivors. About 5,000 pensioners died each year.

There was no corresponding list of the entire membership of the union. There was no information on the smoking habits of union members, pensioned or otherwise. The death certificate for dead pensioners included cause of death, and the address and name of a relative.

Within the union, there were five principal occupations: (1) long-distance drivers, (2) short-distance drivers, (3) dockworkers, (4) truck mechanics, and (5) others outside the trucking industry.

The union had no information about the levels of exposure to diesel fumes. The investigators assumed, however, that those who worked outside the trucking industry were generally not exposed, while those who worked in the industry were exposed.

QUESTION 2a. Given the above information, what would be the best study design possible (cross-sectional, cohort, case-control, proportional mortality) for studying the association of lung cancer and diesel fumes in this population? Keep in mind the need to control for cigarette smoking.

QUESTION 2b. What information is noticeably lacking for such a study?

A two-part study was begun. The first part was an epidemiologic study, while the second was an industrial-hygiene study of the current levels of exposure to diesel exhaust within the trucking industry. While current exposure levels were of great interest, they did not relate directly to the epidemiologic study, in which the exposure of interest occurred many years before. Therefore, the epidemiologic data were analyzed separately from the industrial-hygiene data. This chapter concerns only the epidemiologic data.

The epidemiologic study was a case-control study, in which the cases were all pensioners who had died of lung cancer in the years 1982–1983 (the most recent data available). The controls were a similar number (randomly chosen) of pensioners who had died of causes other than lung cancer, excluding deaths from motor vehicle accidents or bladder cancer.

Information about cigarette smoking was to be obtained from next of kin, via written questionnaires sent by mail. Information about work history was to be obtained from two sources: Teamster records and the next-of-kin interviews. Deaths to be studied were restricted to 1982–1983 because it was felt a sufficient sample size could be obtained with only two years of data. Investigators anticipated 1,000 lung cancer deaths for these two years (10% of the 10,000 total deaths).

QUESTION 3a. Without environmental data indicating the level of exposure to diesel fumes among the study population, what could the definition of exposed and nonexposed be for this study?

QUESTION 3b. Given the definition of "exposure" from part (a) above, how would contingency tables (2 × 2 tables for disease/nondiseased, exposed/nonexposed) be constructed to analyze these data?

QUESTION 3c. Given the data layout in parts (a) and (b), what further steps should be taken to control for the effects of possibly confounding variables, such as age? What statistics might be calculated?

QUESTION 3d. Why were deaths from motor vehicle accidents and bladder cancer excluded from the control series?

The Teamsters work history of the pensioners provided information about whether a man worked as a long-haul or short-haul driver, but not whether he drove a diesel or gasoline truck. Generally, long-haul trucks were diesel while short-haul (until recently) were gasoline. On the other hand, next of kin *were* able to provide information about the type of truck (diesel or gasoline) driven by the decedent (assuming he was a truck driver).

Recall that the questionnaires were to be sent to the next of kin by mail, and returned by mail. Follow-up phone calls were used only if the next of kin failed to respond, or to clarify information that was not clear in a returned questionnaire.

QUESTION 4a. What kind of response rate (rate of participation) would you expect for the next of kin? What do you think would be the lowest possible acceptable response rate?

QUESTION 4b. Do you think the information supplied by the next of kin regarding work history and smoking will be reliable?

QUESTION 4c. What alternatives to a mailed questionnaire were available for data collection from next of kin? What are the advantages and disadvantages of these alternatives?

Because the investigators had two sources of work history (the Teamsters work history and the next-of-kin interviews), they decided to do two different analyses. For each analysis, each man was assigned the occupation in which he had worked the longest.

In the analysis based on Teamsters data, the exposed occupations were long-haul driver, short-haul driver, mechanic, and dockworker. In addition, men outside the trucking industry were divided between those with some potential diesel exhaust (for example, men who worked in service stations or bus drivers), and those unlikely to have had any occupational exposure to diesel fumes (for example, dairy workers). A "sub-analysis" of these data considered as exposed only those who had worked in exposed jobs after 1960, the approximate date when diesel engines were introduced into the trucking fleet.

In the analysis based on next-of-kin data, exposed occupations were truck drivers of predominantly diesel trucks, truck drivers of predominantly gas trucks, truck drivers who drove both types of truck, mechanic, and dockworker. The nonexposed in this analysis were the same men considered nonexposed in the analysis based on the Teamsters data—i.e., those outside the trucking industry with no likely exposure to diesel fumes.

In both analyses, the exposed men were divided according to the duration of work in an exposed job, to determine if increased duration led to increased risk of lung cancer (a kind of dose-response analysis). In both analyses, the investigators controlled for possible confounding by other variables (e.g., smoking).

QUESTION 5a. Define a "confounder."

QUESTION 5b. How do you decide before a study whether a variable is likely to act as a confounder?

QUESTION 5c. How do you decide after data collection whether a variable is acting as a confounder?

QUESTION 5d. Possible confounding by age has already been mentioned. What other possible confounders should be suspect? Can data about these confounders be obtained from either the Teamsters or the next of kin?

In the analysis, there were three variables that were confounders. Each variable was categorized into several levels, making it likely that when the data were stratified for all three confounders simultaneously some strata would have very little data. While it was possible to do stratified analyses with Mantel-Haenszel odds ratios, in such a situation it is common to use a mathematical model (e.g., logistic regression) to estimate a summary odds ratio after adjustment for confounders. Logistic regression also permits the use of continuous predictor variables and allows for the rapid evaluation of interactions between variables. For these reasons, the investigators used logistic regression to do the analysis. Briefly, logistic regression presumes a mathematical model for the relationship between exposure (and other confounders) and disease (the outcome). It is similar to linear regression, but the outcome variable is either 0 or 1 (nondiseased or diseased), while in linear regression the outcome variable is a continuous variable. Although logistic regression was used in the analysis, it is worth noting that it is usually valuable to also conduct at least some stratified analyses via contingency tables. Each investigator needs to have a "feel" for their data prior to using mathematical models available through statistical packages.

Results

Investigators first tested possible confounding factors such as cigarette smoking, pipe/cigar smoking, age, asbestos exposure, diet (vegetable consumption), place of residence, coffee consumption, and prior work in shipyards. Of these, only cigarettes, age, and asbestos acted as confounding variables. No variable appeared to modify the effect of exposure (no interaction terms were necessary). In the final model, variables for cigarette smoking, age, and asbestos exposure were retained in the model along with the exposure variable.

Table 6.1 presents some results based on the Teamsters work history. For full results, see the report by Steenland et al. (1990). Results for the exposed job categories based on work history from next of kin were similar to results based on work history from the Teamsters Union (Table 6.1), and are not presented here.

QUESTION 6a. What is the unadjusted odds ratio for long-haul drivers?

QUESTION 6b. Do these results indicate that the adjustment for potential confounders was worthwhile?

QUESTION 6c. Are any of the adjusted odds ratios in Table 6.1 significantly different from 1.0?

TABLE 6.1 Results Based on Teamsters Work History

	Number	Years Worked	Odds Ratio* (95% CI)
Cases			
Long-haul drivers	609	24	1.27 (0.83–1.93)
Short-haul drivers	121	23	1.31 (0.81–2.11)
Mechanics	50	22	1.69 (0.92–3.09)
Dockworkers	70	23	0.92 (0.55–1.55)
Other, possible diesel exposure	99	—	1.44 (0.88–2.39)
Other, no diesel exposure	45	—	—
Controls			
Long-haul drivers	628	24	
Short-haul drivers	143	24	
Mechanics	37	23	
Dockworkers	94	23	
Other, possible diesel exposure	108	—	
Other, no diesel exposure	75	—	

*Odds ratios were adjusted for age, cigarettes, asbestos exposure, and likely exposure to diesel fumes in jobs not in the trucking industry. Men in jobs in the transport industry were compared to men with no diesel exposure in calculating the odds ratios.

TABLE 6.2 Cases and Controls by Smoking Status

	Never-Smoked	Light Smoker	Heavy Smoker	Former Smoker
Cases				
Long-haul driver	46	108	270	120
Nonexposed	6	13	25	7
Controls				
Long-haul driver	175	87	264	141
Nonexposed	32	11	31	17
Total	259	219	590	285

QUESTION 6d. What would be a further logical step in the analysis of these data?

Table 6.2 presents some data for long-haul drivers and the nonexposed group according to smoking habit. The actual raw data have been altered somewhat for the purpose of this exercise.

QUESTION 7a. For Table 6.2, what is the common odds ratio for long-haul drivers, across all categories of smokers, estimated via the Mantel-Haenszel formula?

QUESTION 7b. Is smoking a positive or negative confounder?

QUESTION 7c. Calculate the Mantel-Haenszel chi-square to test for an association, and derive a test-based confidence interval for the odds ratio in part (a) above.

QUESTION 7d. (optional). In the actual analysis, logistic regression was used to control for confounders. Such control over confounders can be achieved in a variety of ways. Course instructors may obtain a data set (LCT.DAT) with 12 variables (2,082 observations) on diskette for this exercise from the author. The data are described in Table 6.5. All the variables in this data set, except for case/control status, are variables for confounders (age and smoking).

Logistic regression is a model in which the log odds of disease are a function of a linear combination of predictor variables. Age is a predictor variable that can be either continuous or categorical. First, using 2 × 2 tables, determine the odds and log odds of disease for those <45, 45–54, 55–64, 65–74, and 75+ years of age. Plot these logs odds versus age. Then conduct a logistic regression in which the single independent

TABLE 6.3 Risk by Duration of Employment after 1959
for Long-Haul Drivers (based on Teamsters work history)

Years of Work after 1960	Odds Ratio (95% CI)	Standard Error of β	Cases	Controls
0	1.00	—	45	75
1–11	1.08 (.68–1.70)	0.23	162	230
12–17	1.41 (.90–2.12)	0.23	228	203
18+	1.55 (.97–2.47)	0.23	213	171

variable AGE is included, and in which the four categorical variables
AGECAT1, AGECAT2, AGECAT3, AGECAT4 are included. Plot the log
odds of disease from these two models. Comment on the results and how
they compare to the log odds calculated by hand from 2 × 2 tables.
Which would be the better way to model age in the logistic regression?
Now try a model in which EVERSM is included alone, versus a model in
which SMK1A, SMK1B, SMK1C, SMK2, and SMK3 are included. Which
model do you think is preferable? Examine and interpret the coefficients
for the second model.

In Tables 6.3 and 6.4, results are presented of an analysis of lung cancer risk
by duration of employment in certain job categories, for each source of work
history data. These data may be seen as a kind of "dose-response" analysis. The
odds ratios in these tables come from the logistic regression model and are
adjusted for confounding. Table 6.3 also gives the frequencies in the raw data.

QUESTION 8a. In Tables 6.3 and 6.4, what is the "dose" and what is the
"response"?

TABLE 6.4 Risk by Duration of Employment
(based on next-of-kin data)

Occupation	Years of Work	Odds Ratio (95% CI)
Diesel truck driver	1–24	1.27 (.70–2.27)
	25–34	1.26 (.74–2.16)
	35+	1.89 (1.04–3.42)
Gasoline truck driver	1–24	1.24 (.73–1.64)
	25–34	1.10 (.67–1.80)
	35+	1.34 (.81–2.20)

QUESTION 8b. Why did the investigators choose to divide the data into three duration categories, and not two or four?

QUESTION 8c. How do you interpret these data? Is there a "dose-response"? Using 6, 14.5, and 20.5 as scores for the duration of employment categories, conduct a test for linear trend for the raw data in Table 6.3 using the Mantel-extension test. Also determine the slope for a linear trend in adjusted odds ratios for the data in Table 6.3. What is the p-value for the test that the slope (β) equals 0? Of these two tests for trend, which is better?

Discussion

The results presented above indicate that several occupations in the union, presumably exposed to diesel fumes, had a slightly elevated risk of lung cancer compared to those in the union who presumably had no occupational exposure to diesel fumes. Perhaps the most important finding is that the risk of lung cancer increased with duration of employment for long-distance truck drivers (considering only employment after 1960), and also for diesel truck drivers. In spite of these positive results, there are important limitations in this study.

QUESTION 9. What is the most important limitation in this study?

QUESTION 10. If diesel exhaust is carcinogenic, and if truck drivers have in fact had a significant exposure, would this study have been likely to show an elevated lung cancer risk, considering the potential latency? Should this study be repeated in five years?

QUESTION 11. It is possible that only smokers in this study had an excess lung cancer risk. How can this question be answered with the data presented in Table 6.2? Is smoking an effect modifier?

Since this study was begun, a number of other reports on diesel-exposed workers have been published, with most studies indicating some increased lung cancer risks for diesel-exposed workers after controlling for smoking. Gustavson et al. (1990) found an excess risk of lung cancer among bus garage workers, Garshick et al. (1987) found an excess risk among diesel-exposed railroad workers, and Boffeta et al. found small excess risks among individuals reporting diesel exposure in a general population cohort study (1988) and a hospital-based case-control study (1990). Mauderly (1991) in a review article has conclude that the epidemiology to date indicates an excess lung cancer risk of 20%–50% with the primary weakness of the studies begina lack of quantitative exposure data.

TABLE 6.5 Format of Raw Data*

Case	Age	Agecat1	Agecat2	Agecat3	Agecat4	Eversm	Smk1a	Smk1b	Smk1c	Smk2	Smk3
0	41	0	0	0	0	1	0	1	0	0	0
0	50	1	0	0	0	1	0	0	1	0	0

Case: 0 for controls, 1 for lung cancers; Age: age in years at time of death; Agecat1: 1 if $45 \leq$ age < 55, 0 otherwise; Agecat2: 1 if $55 \leq$ age < 65, 0 otherwise; Agecat3: 1 if $65 \leq$ age < 75, 0 otherwise; Agecat4: 1 if age ≥ 75, 0 otherwise; Eversm: 1 is ever-smoker, 0 otherwise; Smk1a: 1 if current smoker, amount unknown, 0 otherwise; Smk1b: 1 if current smoker, 1 pack or less per day, 0 otherwise; Smk1c: 1 if current smoker, more than a pack a day, 0 otherwise; Smk2: 1 if former smoker, quit in last 20 years, 0 otherwise; Smk3: 1 if former smoker, quit 20 or more years ago, 0 otherwise.

*The complete data set is too large to be included in the text (n = 2082), but course instructors may obtain it on diskette from the author.

References

Boffeta P, Stellman s, Garfinkel L. Diesel exhaust exposure and mortality among males in the American Cancer Society prospective study. Am J Ind Med 14: 403–415, 1988.

Boffeta P, Harris R, Wynder E. Case-control study on occupational exposure to diesel exhaust and lung cancer risk. Am J Ind Med 15: 577–591, 1990.

Garshick E, Schenker M, Munoz A, et al. A case-control study of lung cancer on diesel exhaust exposure in railroad workers. Am Rev Respir Dis 135: 1242–1248, 1987.

Gustavson P, Plato N, Lindstrom E, et al. Lung cancer and exposure to diesel exhaust among bus garage workers. Scand J Work Environ Health 16: 348–354, 1990.

Hayes R, Thomas T, Silverman D: Lung cancer in motor exhaust-related occupations. Am J Indust Med 16:685–695, 1989.

Howe G, Fraser D, Lindsay J, et al.: Cancer mortality in relation to diesel fume and coal exposures in a cohort of retired railway workers. JNCI 6:1015–1019, 1983.

NIOSH, Current Intelligence Bulletin #50, DHSS (NIOSH) publication No. 88-116, 1988).

McLaughlin K, Dietz E, Mehl E, et al.: Reliability of surrogate information of cigarette smoking by type of informant. Am J Epidemiol 126:144–146, 1987.

Schenker M, Smith T, Munoz A, et al.: Diesel exposures and mortality among railway workers: results of a pilot study. Br J Indust Med 41:320–327, 1984.

Steenland K, Silverman D, Hornung R: Case-control study of lung cancer and truck driving in the Teamsters Union. Am J Pub Health 80,6:670–674, 1990.

ANSWERS

ANSWER 1. In the United States diesel motors were introduced at the end of the 1950s in the railroad industry, the transport industry (buses and trucks), the construction industry (heavy-equipment vehicles), and in some metal mines. Diesel engines had been introduced even earlier in the shipping industry. Diesel engines were not used in many coal mines until the late 1970s. Miners probably have had the highest exposures because of their work in confined spaces. However, they are difficult to study epidemiologically, because of the relatively small number of exposed in each workplace and the difficulty of determining who is or was exposed at each mine. In addition, the exposure of coal miners, the largest group of exposed miners, is fairly recent and lacks sufficient latency for a lung cancer effect to be observed. Railroad workers had already been studied. Heavy-equipment operators and bus drivers were less numerous than truck drivers. Truck drivers were chosen as the study population.

ANSWER 2a. A cross-sectional design is a poor candidate for a debilitating disease such as lung cancer. A retrospective cohort mortality study of pensioners was a possibility. The referent group could have been either the United States population or Teamsters outside the trucking industry, presumably not exposed to diesel fumes. However, smoking information would be needed, which would be very expensive to obtain for a large cohort. A large cohort would be needed to obtain a sufficient number of lung cancer deaths.

The most feasible study, within the constraints of the time and money of the investigators, was a case-control study in which the cases were pensioners who had died recently. The Teamsters union could identify such men and had death certificates and work history for them already in hand. Smoking information and further work history information could be obtained from next of kin. To make the quality of information on smoking and work history comparable, it was decided to also use dead controls, randomly chosen from those who did not die of lung cancer. Deaths from motor vehicle accidents and bladder cancer, both associated with truck driving, were also excluded.

A case-control study in which cases and controls are dead is a study of the same population as would be studied in a proportionate mortality study, although the analysis differs and the case-control study may exclude some causes from the control group. The case-control analysis is generally preferable, especially if there is an internal nonexposed group (see the Introduction to Part II.)

ANSWER 2b. Information on the level of exposure to diesel fumes of study subjects.

ANSWER 3a. Without data on exposure to diesel fumes, investigators could still compare the risk of lung cancer risk of the five principal occupations in the Teamsters union (long-haul driver, short-haul driver, mechanic, dockworker, and those outside the trucking industry). It was presumed that those outside the trucking industry had no occupational exposure to diesel exhaust. Hence, there would be four "exposed" groups and one "nonexposed" group.

ANSWER 3b. Given the definition of exposure above, four sets of 2 × 2 contingency tables would be set up in which the exposed would be long-haul drivers, short-haul drivers, mechanics, and dockworkers. In each case the nonexposed would be the same group of men outside the trucking industry, as shown below for long-haul drivers and mechanics.

	Cases	Controls	Odds Ratio
Long-haul truckers (exp)	a	b	
Outside trucking industry (nonexp)	c	d	ad/bc
Mechanic (exp)	a'	b'	
Outside trucking industry (nonexp)	c	d	a'd/b'c

ANSWER 3c. Further steps to control confounding would typically involve stratification by levels of possible confounders, such as age, followed by calculation of the Mantel-Haenszel summary odds ratio, and the corresponding chi-square test of significance or 95% confidence intervals. Modeling (logistic regression) might also be used to control confounding.

ANSWER 3d. In a case-control study, the controls should represent the same population from which cases arise, but be free of disease. The purpose of the control population is to estimate the proportion of exposed among those free of disease, to compare to the proportion among the diseased. Here deaths from bladder cancer and motor vehicle accidents were excluded from the control group because truck drivers may die more frequently of these causes, and hence the proportion of truck drivers (exposed) in the controls would have been somewhat greater than appropriate, resulting in an artificial decrease in the odds ratio. Using the same reasoning, for example, the investigators who originally studied the association of lung cancer and smoking excluded from the control series people with diseases associated with smoking, such as bronchitis and emphysema.

ANSWER 4a. In this study the investigators were able to find next of kin of 80% of the deceased study subjects. Of those found, virtually all agreed to be interviewed. There is no minimal acceptable percentage, but as a general rule 70–80% participation should be a reasonable goal. A participation rate less than 50% is a cause for serious concern. Sometimes it is possible to determine if the nonparticipants are similar to the participants with respect to demographic variables such as age, race, and sex, lending some reassurance that the participants are representative of the target population. However, the key variable of interest is exposure, and typically no data are available for exposure for nonparticipants.

ANSWER 4b. There are studies that indicate that the smoking information from next of kin regarding the decedent is relatively trustworthy, although it loses validity when more detail is required (such as age when smoking began) (McLaughlin et al., 1987). The situation for work history is similar. The information from the union regarding work history for this study was quite detailed and trustworthy because the union required good documentation of at least twenty years of work history before awarding a pension. Pensions involved a considerable amount of money, so both the union and individual Teamsters were usually quite systematic in documenting work history.

ANSWER 4c. Alternatives to mailed interviews followed by phone interviews for nonrespondents were (1) phone interviews without any prior mailing or (2) person-to-person interviews. Each is more expensive than mailed interviews followed by some phone calls, but each yields better information. As always in observational studies such as this, there is a trade-off between the quality of information and what is feasible within budget constraints.

ANSWER 5a. A confounder is a variable other than the exposure variable that is associated with both the exposure and the disease. A confounder can distort the measurement of the association between the exposure variable and the disease, unless the investigator controls its effects via stratification (or via modeling).

ANSWER 5b. Before the study, the investigator can identify potential confounders from a review of the epidemiologic literature to discover known risk factors for disease. If these variables differ among exposure groups they will act as confounders. Age, race, and sex are usually potential confounders. It is important during data collection to gather information on such potential confounders.

ANSWER 5c. After data collection, investigators can test whether a variable is actually acting as a confounder by testing whether control of such a confounder changes the measure of association between disease and exposure.

ANSWER 5d. In a study of lung cancer, confounders other than age would be race, smoking, diet (consumption of vitamin A or retinoids), and asbestos exposure. Data on all these variables were available primarily from next of kin.

ANSWER 6a. The unadjusted odds ratio is (609)(75)/(45)(628) = 1.62.

ANSWER 6b. The odds ratio adjusted for confounders is 1.27, which indicates that other variables were indeed acting as confounders.

ANSWER 6c. None of the odds ratios differs significantly from 1.0, but there is a pattern of elevated odds ratios for most occupations within the trucking industry.

ANSWER 6d. A logical next step would be an evaluation of lung cancer risk by duration of employment in an occupation of interest ("dose-response").

ANSWER 7a. The common odds ratio (Mantel-Haenszel) is 1.36.

ANSWER 7b. The crude odds ratio for Table 6.2 was 1.46, while the odds ratio adjusted for smoking was 1.36. Smoking is a positive confounder.

ANSWER 7c. For the data above, the chi-square statistic is 2.57, with one degree of freedom. The probability that such a statistic would have occurred by chance, under the null hypothesis of no association between long-haul driving and lung cancer, is approximately 11%. The 95% test-based confidence interval is (0.93, 1.97). Note that this range of plausible values includes 1.0. The width of the confidence interval is a function of sample size, and it is possible that a large sample would have yielded the same odds ratio (1.36) with a narrower confidence interval.

ANSWER 7d. Using 2 × 2 tables the log odds of disease for the five age categories are −1.11, 0.07, 0.13, .05, and −0.78. The odds go up and then come down with age, in an upside down U-shaped pattern. This is a reflection of the proportion of lung cancer deaths among all deaths, which is low initially, increases with age, and then drops back down at older ages. A logistic model with AGE as a continuous variable yields a negative coefficient. Plotting the log odds as a function of age yields a straight line with a downward slope. Use of the categorical or dummy variables AGECAT1–AGECAT4 (under age 45 is the referent group and has a 0 for all of these variables) in the model yields exactly the same log odds as seen in the 2 × 2 tables (e.g., for AGECAT4 the coefficient is 0.3209, with an intercept of −1.0986, yielding a log odds of −0.78). The point here is that use of continuous variable for age may be misleading, because it assumes that the log odds decreases monotonically with age.

The model with AGE does not fit the data very well, while the model with the categorical variables for age makes no assumption about the shape of the curve relating the log odds of disease and age. The categorical variables for age would be preferable here. An alternative would be to use a quadratic term (age squared) in addition to the variable AGE.

Regarding smoking, remember that the data on smoking comes from the next of kin. The next of kin generally could remember whether the decedent was a current smoker, but sometimes could not remember the amount smoked. Hence, there are considerable missing data on amount smoked. These missing data may be "modeled" by including a dichotomous variable for "current smoker, missing amount" (SMK1A). Note that unless the missing smoking data are included in the model, observations without amount-smoked data would have to be dropped from the analysis.

An alternative method of modeling smoking is to use "pack-years," but this has the disadvantage that next of kin have to remember not only amount smoked but duration of smoking. Use of pack-years in this data set resulted in missing values for 25% of the population.

Both the single variable EVERSM and the set of variables SMK1A, SMK1B, SMK1C, SMK2, and SMK3 are strong predictors. The likelihood ratio statistic is slightly more significant with the set of five smoking variables, but the main reason that the set of five is to be preferred is that the use of the ever-never variable (EVERSM) is tantamount to stratifying the data by only two smoking categories. This may allow residual confounding by smoking within the large stratum of ever-smokers. Use of five smoking categories is preferable because it is likely to control confounding better. Use of SMK1A, SMK1B, SMK1C, SMK2, SMK3 yields estimated odds ratios versus the referent category (never-smokers, with values of 0 for all five of these variables) of 7.2, 6.5, 9.9, 5.0, 2.6. These odds ratios make reasonable sense. Current smokers with missing data on amount smoked (7.2) are in between light current smokers (6.5) and heavy current smokers (9.9), while former smokers have lower odds ratios, decreasing with increasing years since quitting.

ANSWER 8a. Here the "dose" is duration of employment in an occupation exposed to diesel fumes (the ideal "dose" would be the cumulative exposure to diesel exhaust received by each study participant). The response is death from lung cancer.

ANSWER 8b. A dose-response is usually evaluated in categorical data by observing that there is an increasing linear trend in risk with increasing level of exposure. Here risk is measured by the odds ratio, while the exposure level is the number of years worked in a certain job. The linear trend may be assessed via a weighted linear regression of the odds ratios, with the weights dependent on the sample size of each category (alternatively, one may test for a linear trend in proportions in the raw data via the Mantel-extension test). The investigator usually seeks to have approximately equal numbers of study subjects in each exposure category, so the variance of the data (odds ratios) for each category is about equal. The investigator also seeks to have at least three categories so as to be able to assess a trend, but not so many categories that there are only a small number of study subjects in each category, leading to instability (wide variance in the odds ratios). Here the investigators chose three categories of duration, each with approximately the same numbers of subjects.

An alternative to this type of dose-response analysis is to use a single continuous variable for duration in a model, such as logistic regression (no categories). The test of significance of the coefficient for this variable, resulting from the logistic regression, would signify whether there was a significant trend in risk with increasing duration.

ANSWER 8c. There does appear to be a positive trend in lung cancer risk with increased duration of employment as either a long-haul driver or a driver of diesel trucks. A test for a linear trend in the raw data via the Mantel-extension test yields a chi-square statistic (one degree of freedom) of $360,202/15,403 = 23.3$, which is highly significant (p less than 0.01). A test for a linear trend in the adjusted odds ratio from logistic regression yields a slope (β) of .026 with a standard error of .013. A test of significance of this slope yields a Z-statistic of 2.00, with a p-value of approximately .05. The latter test is the more appropriate test for trend because it is based on odds ratios that have been adjusted for confounders.

Other occupations are not shown in Tables 6.3 and 6.4 because they did not show a positive trend. Furthermore, no such positive trend was observed for long-haul drivers unless only their employment after 1960 (the approximate introduction of diesel engines) was considered.

ANSWER 9. The most important limitation to the data presented here is the lack of information on exposure to diesel fumes. Subsequently, data from the industrial hygiene survey of *current* exposures (Zaebst et al., 1991) indicated that truck drivers are exposed to diesel exhaust at levels about the same as ambient levels on the highway. These in turn are about double the background exposures in urban air. It is possible that earlier exposures for drivers were higher due to cabs leaking exhaust (the exhaust pipe used to be underneath the cab), lack of air-conditioning, and other changes in fuel and engines. The survey also revealed that mechanics had the highest current levels of diesel exposure, while dockworkers using propane-powered forklifts had the lowest. Note that the risk of mechanics is highest in Table 6.1, while the risk of dock-workers was lowest. Mechanics, however, did not show consistent increased risk with increased duration of employment.

While the current exposure data appeared generally consistent with the epidemiologic findings (Steenland et al., 1992), historical levels of diesel exposure (the most relevant for the epidemiologic study) were not available.

Other important limitations are possible errors in classification of smoking habits or work history by next of kin. In general, misclassification errors for work history (exposure), assuming cases and controls were equally misclassified, would bias findings toward the null hypothesis. Misclassification of a confounder such as smoking could have a variety of effects (see Kupper, 1984).

ANSWER 10. Under the assumption that diesel exhaust may act as a tumor initiator, the maximum period of potential latency is relatively short for lung cancer in this study (first exposures in 1960 at the earliest, lung cancers observed in 1982–1983). Many solid tumors require more than 20 years latency. Therefore, it would be worth repeating the study in five years. If diesel exhaust is carcinogenic, it might act as a promoter rather than an initiator, in which case the limited potential latency discussed above would be irrelevant. If this were the case, one might expect to see a lung cancer effect only in smokers (see Answer 11 below).

ANSWER 11. It is always difficult to determine the risk for never-smokers versus smokers in studies of lung cancer because lung cancer is very uncommon for never-smokers, limiting any power to observe risks in this category. However, the hypothetical data in Table 6.2 would suggest no effect modification. The odds ratio for nonsmokers is 1.40, while the odds ratio for never-smokers (all other categories combined) is 1.33. These data would indicate that long-haul driving has the same strength as a risk factor for lung cancer among smokers and nonsmokers. A similar observation was made in the actual data.

References for Answers

Kupper L. Effects of the use of unreliable surrogate variables on the validity of epidemiologic research studies. Am J Epidemiol 120: 643–648, 1984.

Steenland K, Silverman D, Zaebst D. Exposure to diesel exhaust in the trucking industry and possible relationships with lung cancer. Am J Ind Med (in press), 1992.

Zaebst D, Clapp D, Blade L, Marlow D, Steenland K, Hornung R, Scheutzle D, Butler J. Quantitative determination of trucking industry workers' exposure to diesel exhaust particles. Am Ind Hyg Assoc J 52, 21: 529–541, 1991.

Chapter 7 | Silica and Lung Cancer: A Proportionate Mortality Study

KYLE STEENLAND

Animal studies in the late 1970s and early 1980s showed that crystalline silica (quartz) could promote and induce lung tumors (Stettler et al., 1984). It was therefore of interest to determine whether silica-exposed human populations were at an increased risk of lung cancer.

A second hypothesis of interest was whether those who have silicosis, a fibrotic disease of the lung, were at increased risk of lung cancer. It has been hypothesized that some aspect of silicosis, such as enzymes released by macrophages that are destroyed in the silicotic process, induces lung cancer (Goldsmith et al., 1982).

In order to investigate these hypotheses, NIOSH investigators sought to find a cohort of workers exposed primarily to silica. Silica exposure in the workplace principally occurs among foundry workers, miners, granite workers, and sandblasters.

QUESTION 1. Speculate on advantages and disadvantages of a cohort study of these potential cohorts.

QUESTION 2. Is a case-control study based in the general population a possible alternative for studying the association of lung cancer and silica exposure?

Materials and Methods

Researchers chose to study granite cutters organized in the Granite Cutters Union. These men worked in granite sheds near quarries and cut granite to make gravestones, building material, etc. They had historically been exposed to very high levels of silica, without any potentially confounding exposures. Historical dust levels were approximately 20–50 million particles per cubic foot (mppcf) through the 1940s, but were lowered to approximately 3–5 mppcf thereafter, after it was recognized that high levels of silica dust caused silicosis. Silicosis, which had been very common among granite cutters, became much rarer after dust levels were lowered. The Granite Cutters Union had records of deaths among its members, but not a list of all its members over time. Death records went back in time to January 1, 1949, and continued until the early 1980s. The union paid death benefits (the amount determined by duration of union membership) to families of decedents, so next of kin had a financial incentive to inform the union of deaths.

QUESTION 3. What kind of study could be done in this situation? What group would be the nonexposed comparison population? What are the potential disadvantages of such a study?

Union records enabled the identification of 2,274 deaths. Last name, date of death, and the state in which the decedent had worked were available from death records, but Social Security number was not. Death certificates were obtained for 1,911 of these individuals (84%), of whom 1,905 were white males. Six men were missing age at death, and analyses were restricted to 1899 white males for whom age at death was known. For 90% of the records, the amount of funeral money awarded (corresponding to length of union membership) was also available.

A proportionate mortality analysis was performed, comparing the granite cutters to the U.S. population. Deaths were stratified by age and calendar time to avoid confounding from these variables. The proportion of deaths from lung cancer, out of all deaths, in the exposed cohort versus the U.S. population was calculated. A proportionate cancer mortality ratio (PCMR) was also calculated for lung cancer, and a mortality odds ratio (MOR) was also calculated by treating the data as if they were case-control data.

QUESTION 4. With 16% of the deaths missing due to lack of death certificates, should researchers have proceeded with the study or stopped because they could not be sure the known deaths were representative of all deaths? What steps were possible to assure that the known deaths were in fact representative?

Analyses of the 1,905 deaths in the study population revealed that the majority died in Vermont (36%), followed by New York (17%), and Massachusetts (14%). Seventy-one percent of the study population had been union members for at least 20 years. The average age at death was 69, and the average year of death was 1962. A comparison of those with death certificates and those without revealed little or no difference regarding age at death, state of death, and year of death.

Results

Full results from this study may be found in Steenland et al. (1986).
Table 7.1 gives the results from some of the most important causes of interest.

QUESTION 5. How were the "expecteds" calculated in Table 7.1? Why
have the PMRs in Table 7.1 have been "standardized" for age and
calendar time. What does this mean?

Much of the large tuberculosis excess in Table 7.1 was due to silicotuberculosis.
In past decades, silicosis was frequently labeled silicotuberculosis (the two
diseases have much in common histologically), whereas in recent years silicosis
has generally been separated from tuberculosis and grouped with other pneumoconioses. Most of the excess in nonmalignant respiratory disease seen in
Table 7.1 was due to silicosis as well. Lung cancer shows a slight excess of
borderline statistical significance. Heart disease shows an expected deficit due
to the healthy worker effect.

The problem of competing causes, typical of proportionate mortality studies,
is particularly pronounced here not only because of the deficit in heart disease
(typical of working populations when compared to the general population), but
also because of the counterbalancing excesses in tuberculosis and nonmalignant respiratory disease. Therefore, a proportionate cancer mortality ratio
(PCMR) was calculated, which for lung cancer was 1.09 (95% CI 0.89–1.34).
In the PCMR, the proportion of deaths from lung cancer among all *cancer*
deaths was calculated among the granite cutters and compared to the expected
number based on the U.S. white male population. As a further attempt to
eliminate the competing cause problem, a mortality odds ratio (MOR) analysis
was conducted in which the odds of exposure were compared for lung cancer
deaths (cases) versus other cancer deaths that served as controls (Spiegelman et
al., 1983). Controls were restricted to other cancers because other important
causes of death (e.g., heart disease and silicosis) were associated with silica
exposure in this study. The nonexposed group was again U.S. white male
decedents. The population considered in this analysis was the same as in the

TABLE 7.1 Proportionate Mortality Ratios for Selected Causes

Cause	Observed	Expected	PMR	95% Confidence Interval
Tuberculosis	262	19.3	13.56	(11.94–15.27)
Nonmalignant respiratory disease*	183	43.7	4.18	(3.60–4.84)
Lung cancer	97	81.1	1.19	(0.97–1.46)
Heart disease	574	711.3	0.80	(0.74–0.87)

*Excluding bronchitis, pneumonia, and influenza; including emphysema and pneumoconioses.

PCMR analysis above, except that an odds ratio rather than a PMR (risk ratio) was calculated. The odds ratio resulting from this analysis was 1.17 (95% CI 0.94–1.51).

QUESTION 6. Results to this point indicate only a slight elevation of risk of lung cancer for those exposed to silica versus the U.S. population. Can you think of further analyses that would now be appropriate?

Table 7.2 shows results of analyses by years of union membership for lung cancer, tuberculosis, and nonmalignant respiratory disease. PCMR results for lung cancer were similar and are not presented here.

QUESTION 7. Do the data in Table 7.2 support a positive dose-response relationship for lung cancer? What is the relevance of the data for tuberculosis and nonmalignant respiratory disease in this table?

To more formally test for the trend in disease risk by years in the union, it might be preferable (1) to have more than the two points in Table 7.2 (which is restricted to less than 20 years, more than 20 years), and (2) to conduct an internal comparison of those with more years compared to those with fewer years. An internal comparison can be done as a case-control analysis (yielding an MOR), diminishing the competing cause of death problem. An internal comparison also avoids the problem of the healthy worker effect (it also avoids the problem of comparing indirectly standardized measures such as PMRs, see the Appendix for a fuller discussion of this point). By way of example, in Table 7.3 the data are presented for silicosis deaths stratified by three categories of duration of time in the union.

QUESTION 8. Calculate the MH odds ratios for silicosis by increasing years in the union, and the Mantel test for trend (see Appendix). In Table

TABLE 7.2 Analyses by Years of Union Membership

Cause	Observed	PMR	95% Confidence Interval
Lung cancer			
Less than 20 years in union	30	1.33	(0.90–1.91)
20+ years in union	49	1.08	(0.80–1.44)
Tuberculosis			
Less than 20 years in union	72	9.39	(7.35–11.83)
20+ years in union	182	17.07	(14.68–19.74)
Nonmalignant respiratory disease			
Less than 20 years in union	33	3.36	(2.32–4.73)
20+ years in union	137	5.00	(4.20–5.91)

TABLE 7.3 Risk of Death from Silicosis
by Years in the Union

Cause and Age at Death	Years in Union		
	7.5	17.5	30
Age < 60			
Silicosis	43	20	21
Other deaths	187	62	53
Age 60–69			
Silicosis	32	20	115
Other deaths	124	55	162
Age 70+			
Silicosis	15	22	139
Other deaths	88	104	548

7.3, deaths from tuberculosis and pneumoconioses have been combined and are together considered "silicosis" (cases), while other deaths excluding lung cancers serve as the controls. The data have been stratified by three age groups.

The data were also analyzed by year of death, under the assumption that men who died earlier would have worked earlier when exposures were higher. For lung cancer, the PMR for those who died prior to 1960 was 0.98 (27 observed), while it was 1.38 (36 observed) for those who died from 1960 to 1970, and 1.22 (34 observed) for those who died after 1970. This analysis did not indicate that those with presumably higher silica exposures had higher lung cancer rates.

Researchers considered the possibility that the large number of men dying from silicosis might be those with highest silica exposure who in turn might have gone on to develop lung cancer. However, the average age of death for those with any mention of silicosis on their death certificate (excluding those with lung cancer) was 67, while the average age of death of the lung cancers was 66. Therefore it did not seem likely that silicotics dying at an early age were obscuring a later lung cancer risk.

Given that the findings for lung cancer were largely negative, the investigation then focused on whether there was any evidence that men with silicosis had higher lung cancer rates. Unfortunately, from the data available to us (death certificates), it was impossible to determine who had silicosis. As a crude approximation, any man with mention of silicosis on the death certificate was considered a silicotic. A case-control approach was used; cases were the 97 men with lung cancer. The odds of "exposure" (mention of silicosis on the death certificate) for the cases versus controls was calculated.

QUESTION 9. How would you select controls for this case-control study of lung cancer and silicosis?

Analysis of the case-control study found that 26 of the 97 lung cancer cases had a mention of silicosis on the death certificate, while only 14 of the 135 controls did. Cases and controls were similar regarding age at death, number of years of good standing in the union, and year of death.

QUESTION 10. What is the implication of the finding that cases and controls did not differ with respect to age at death, year of death, and time in union? Calculate the odds ratio for silicosis and lung cancer, as well as a confidence interval.

Discussion

This proportionate mortality study has shown a large excess of silicosis in this cohort, indicating heavy exposure to silica. The excess of silicosis increased with duration of union membership. Lung cancer in this cohort showed a slight excess compared to the U.S. comparison population (PMR 1.19). Other analyses (mortality odds ratio, proportionate cancer mortality ratio), designed to correct for competing-cause problems inherent in proportionate mortality studies, yielded similar or less elevated results for lung cancer. Lung cancer did not show an increase with increasing years of union membership. Researchers concluded that there was little evidence that lung cancer in this heavily exposed cohort was associated with silica exposure per se. On the other hand, there was some evidence that silicotics had an excess risk of lung cancer, based on an analysis of contributory causes and significant conditions listed on the death certificate.

There were no smoking data for the cohort, and smoking is a major risk factor for lung cancer. Working populations generally smoke more than the general population, at least since the 1960s. One might be concerned that smoking would act as a positive confounder for lung cancer when the granite cutters were compared to the U.S. population. However, the study was largely negative for lung cancer, obviating the potential worry that a positive finding might be due to confounding by smoking rather than an effect of exposure.

Epidemiologic studies of lung cancer among workers exposed to silica have yielded contradictory results, some being positive and some negative (for example, see Brown et al., 1984; Davis et al., 1983; Merlo et al., 1991). Studies restricted to silicotics, on the other hand, have been virtually all positive for lung cancer, often with markedly elevated rate ratios (Amandus et al., 1991; Chiyotani et al., 1990; Finkelstein et al., 1987; Forastiere et al., 1987; Hessel et al., 1990; Infante-Rivard et al., 1990; Kurppa et al., 1986; Mastrangelo et al., 1988; Merlo et al., 1990; Ny et al., 1990; Schuler et al., 1986; Westerholm et al., 1980; Zambon et al., 1987).

The issue of whether heavy silica exposure leads to lung cancer remains unresolved. While it is possible that some aspect of the silicotic disease process leads to lung cancer (so that silicosis is an intermediate variable on the pathway from exposure to disease), those who get silicosis are usually those with the highest exposure to silica. Lung cancer could simply reflect the higher doses received by silicotics, independently of silicosis.

References

Amandus H, Shy C, Wing S: Silicosis and lung cancer in North Carolina Dusty Trades Workers, Am J Indust Med 20,1:57–70, 1991.

Amandus H, Costello J: Silicosis and lung cancer in U.S. metal miners. Arch Env Health 46,2:82–89, 1991.

Brown D, Kaplan S, Zumwalde R: A retrospective cohort mortality study of goldminers exposed to amphibole mineral and silica. In: Goldsmith D, Winn D, Shy C (eds.), *Silica, Silicosis, and Cancer.* New York: Preager, 1986.

Chiyotani K, Saito K, Okubo T, et al.: Lung cancer risk among pneumoconiosis patients in Japan, with special reference to silicotics. IARC Sci Publ 97:95–104, 1990.

Davis L, Wegman D, Monson R, et al.: Mortality experience of Vermont granite workers. Am J Indust Med 4:705–723, 1984.

Finkelstein M, Liss G, Krammer F, et al.: Mortality among workers receiving compensation awards for silicosis in Ontario 1940–1985. Br J Indust Med 1987, 44:588–594.

Forastiere F, Lagorio S, Michelozzi P, et al.: Silica, silicosis, and lung cancer among ceramic workers: a case-referent study. Am J Indust Med 10:363–370, 1987.

Goldsmith D, Guidotti T, Johnston D: Does occupational exposure to silica cause lung cancer? Am J Indust Med 3:423–440, 1982.

Hessel P, Sluis-Cremer G, Hnizdo E: Silica exposure, silicosis, and lung cancer: a necroscopy study. Br J Indust Med 47:4–9, 1990.

Infante-Rivard C, Armstrong B, Petitclerc M, et al.: Lung cancer mortality and silicosis in Quebec, 1938–85. Lancet (December 23–30):1504–1507, 1990.

Kurppa K, Gudbergsson H, Hannunkari I, et al.: Lung cancer among silicotics in Finland. In: Goldsmith D, Winn D, Shy C (eds.), *Silica, Silicosis, and Cancer.* New York: Preager, 1986.

Mastrangelo G, Zambon P, Simonato L, et al.: A case-referent study investigating the relationship between exposure to silica dust and lung cancer. Int Arch Occup Environ Health 60:299–302, 1988.

Merlo F, Doria M, Fontana L, et al.: Mortality from specific causes among silicotic subjects. IARC Sci Publ 97:105–111, 1990.

Merlo F, Constantini M, Reggiardo G, et al.: Lung cancer risk in silica brick workers. Epidemiol 2,4:299–403, 1991.

Ng T, Chan Shiu, Lee J: Mortality of a cohort of men in a silicosis register: further evidence of an association with lung cancer. Am J Indust Med 17:163–171, 1990.

Schuler G, Ruttner J: Silicosis and lung cancer in Switzerland. In: Goldsmith D, Winn D, Shy C (eds.), *Silica, Silicosis, and Cancer.* New York: Preager, 1986.

Spiegelman D, Wang J, Wegman D: Iterative electronic computing of the mortality odds ratio. Am J Epidemiol 118:599–607, 1983.

Steenland K, Beaumont J: A proportionate mortality study of granite cutters. Am J Indust Med 9:189–201, 1986.

Stettler L, Groth D, Lal J, et al.: Lung tumors in rates treated with quartz and other minerals by intratracheal injection. In: Goldsmith D, Winn D, Shy C (eds.), *Silica, Silicosis, and Lung Cancer*. New York, Praeger, 1986.

Westerholm P: Silicosis, observations on a case register. Scand J Work Environ Health 6 (suppl 2):1–86, 1980.

Zambon P, Simonato L, Mastrangelo G: Mortality of workers compensated for silicosis during the period 1959–1963 in the Veneto region of Italy. Scand J Work Environ Health 13:118–123, 1987.

ANSWERS

ANSWER 1. The main disadvantage of a cohort study of foundry workers and miners is that they are often exposed to other known lung carcinogens. Foundry workers are exposed to polycyclic aromatic hydrocarbons (PAHs), and miners are often exposed to radon daughters. Miners also may not be exposed to appreciable levels of silica, depending on the ore they are mining. Sandblasters have the advantage that they are exposed to very high levels of silica (sand is mostly silica, and sandblasting creates large amounts of respirable dust), but the disadvantage that they do not work within a single industry and it is difficult to assemble a large cohort with good records. Granite workers are the best candidate. Granite workers are exposed to high levels of silica (granite is approximately 10–30% silica), granite workers have few other exposures, and they are organized in an industry centered around granite quarries.

ANSWER 2. Silica exposure is rare in the general population; therefore, a case-control study based in the general population is probably not a good study design. A case-control study based in the general population would have to be conducted within a population in which silica-exposure was prevalent. One possibility would be a population-based case-control study in an area in which work in granite quarries was common.

ANSWER 3. When the study population is limited to decedents, a traditional cohort study with person-time denominators is not possible, because the population at risk over time is not known. In this situation, it is possible to do a proportionate mortality study, in which the proportions of deaths due to the cause of interest are compared between the exposed and nonexposed study groups, yielding a proportionate mortality ratio (PMR).

Proportionate mortality studies have the disadvantage that the proportions of death due to one cause are not independent of the proportion of death due to another cause (see part II Introduction for a discussion). For example, if the nonexposed comparison population were the U.S. population, due to the healthy worker effect one would expect a deficit in the relative proportion of heart disease deaths among the granite cutters, and a corresponding increase in the proportion of deaths due to cancer. It is possible to partly or completely avoid this problem of competing causes in proportionate mortality studies through several methods, such as (1) choosing a working population as the nonexposed comparison group, (2) conducting proportionate cancer mortality analyses (PCMR) among all cancer deaths, and (3) analyzing the same data as if it were a case-control study. This last approach results in an odds ratio (Miettenen and Wang, 1981), and is sometimes called a mortality odds ratio analysis (MOR). For the granite cutters, researchers used methods (2) and (3) above, in addition to a traditional PMR analysis.

Among the granite cutters there was no clearly defined "no exposure" or "very low-exposure" subgroup within the total exposed cohort, making an internal comparison difficult. Under these circumstances, the U.S. population was used as the nonexposed comparison population.

Aside from the analytical problems stemming from of the proportionate mortality design, it is important that known deaths be a complete listing of all deaths or at least a representative sample. If the known deaths are a biased sample, in which some causes are overrepresented compared to the underlying population, results will also be biased. In this study, the union believed it had a relatively complete list of deaths because of the fairly strong financial incentive for next of kin to report deaths. Death payments were in the range of $100–$300, which in the period when most deaths occurred (the 1940s to the 1960s) represented a considerable sum of money.

ANSWER 4. There is no golden rule about what size sample is likely to be representative. However, 84% is a high percentage. Without any prior belief that the 84% sample of deaths was skewed in favor of some causes of death versus others, there is a good chance that the sample was representative. Random chance alone is unlikely to result in such a large proportion of deaths not being an accurate reflection of the total. As a check, researchers analyzed the age at death, year of death, and state of death for those for whom they had death certificates compared to those for whom they did not. While comparability for these variables could not assure that underlying causes of death were distributed similarly among those with and without death certificates, at least comparability would assure that both groups were similar demographically, making it less likely that they would have a different pattern of cause of death.

ANSWER 5. The "expecteds" represent the number of deaths from a given cause expected among the granite cutters if the proportions of death from different causes in the cohort were the same as among deaths of U.S. white males of the same age and during the same calendar time. Standardization for age and calendar time is done as a means of controlling for confounding. The deaths in both granite cutters and U.S. white males were stratified by five-year age and calendar time at death strata. The proportion of all deaths in each stratum among U.S. white males due to a particular cause—say, lung cancer—was then multiplied by the number of deaths in that stratum among granite cutters to obtain the expected deaths from lung cancer among granite cutters in that stratum. Then observed and expected deaths for all age and calendar time strata were summed to obtain the overall observed and expected numbers shown in Table 7.1.

ANSWER 6. An attempt to evaluate a dose-response is in order now. No data on actual dose are available. However, men could be grouped by duration of union membership, which was available for approximately 90% of the study population. Years of union membership, in what was traditionally a highly organized trade, could be considered a rough approximation to duration of exposure. Duration of exposure, in turn, may be considered a rough approximation of cumulative dose.

ANSWER 7. The data do not support a positive dose-response for lung cancer. The analyses for tuberculosis and nonmalignant respiratory disease do show an increase with increasing years of union membership. Since these causes are clearly related to silica, results by years of union membership for these causes lends validity to the assumption that increasing years of union membership correlates with increasing exposure to silica.

ANSWER 8. The chi-square (one degree of freedom) is $(759.2)^2/25,099$ = 22.96, which indicates a highly significant trend of increasing risk of silicosis by increasing years in the union. The MH odds ratios are 1.00, 1.36, and 2.05 for 7.5, 17.5, and 30 years in the union.

ANSWER 9. There were many ways to select controls. The purpose of the controls was to provide a representative sample of the "base" or underlying population who did not develop lung cancer and did not die of other causes associated with silica exposure. Here the underlying population is deceased granite cutters. One method would be to choose a random sample of men who did not die of lung cancer or silicosis. Researchers were concerned, however, that silicosis would go unmentioned on the death certificate for many men. It was assumed that for most cases of lung cancer, physicians would have read chest X rays, noted any silicosis, and listed it on the death certificate. Hence, for the lung cancer cases, researchers believed the death certificate would provide a reasonable estimate of who had silicosis. To provide a comparable set of controls, regarding the completeness of silicosis ascertainment on the death certificate, other cancer deaths were chosen. Cancer cases are usually hospitalized and chest X rays are usually ordered routinely to detect possible metastases. Researchers chose 135 men who died of eight cancer sites (stomach, colon, rectum, pancreas, liver, bladder, brain).

ANSWER 10. The fact that cases and controls do not differ by age, year of death, or length of union membership implies that these variables are not confounders, and the odds ratio calculated from a simple single contingency table will suffice. The odds ratio for these data is (121)(26)/(71)(14), or 3.16. The chi-square test of association yields a chi-square of 10.68, and the 95% test-based confidence interval for the odds ratio is (1.58, 6.30).

References for Answers

Miettinen O, Wang J: An alternative to the proportionate mortality ratio. Am J Epidemiol 114:144–148, 1981.

Part III | Cross-Sectional Studies

Cross-sectional studies, or prevalence studies, ascertain exposure and disease in a given population at the same time. For example, an investigator may study the prevalence of low birthweight by race among newborns at a given hospital. The investigator can then determine the prevalence of disease (e.g., low birthweight) among the exposed (e.g., nonwhites) compared to the nonexposed (e.g., whites).

The simultaneous ascertainment of exposure and disease creates one of the principal difficulties in cross-sectional studies, the determination of whether the exposure preceded the disease. For example, suppose the investigator studies the prevalence of genetic abnormalities in workers exposed to a pesticide and in a referent group, and finds a higher prevalence in those exposed to the pesticide. It is possible that the genetic abnormalities existed in the peripheral lymphocytes of these workers prior to their exposure to the pesticide, due to genetic factors which by chance occur more frequently in the pesticide-exposed workers than the referents.

Sometimes it is even possible that the "outcome" may have caused the exposure, rather than the other way around. For example, suppose investigators find that the level of dioxin in the serum of Air Force personnel who served in Vietnam is higher in diabetics than in nondiabetics. It is possible that dioxin leads to diabetes, but it is also possible that diabetes causes a metabolic disorder that causes more dioxin to be released from the body fat into the bloodstream.

Cross-sectional studies are most appropriate for diseases or conditions that are of sufficiently long course and not drastically debilitating. Any disease that causes disability and withdrawal from the work force is less likely to be detected among those currently exposed. A decrease in lung function might be a good candidate for a cross-sectional study, but cancer would not be. A cross-sectional study of carpal tunnel syndrome may miss those severe cases that have had to leave the work force, thus distorting the measurement of exposure-disease association.

Despite these problems of prevalence studies, they are commonly done and often yield valuable information. They frequently are less expensive than cohort or case-control studies of disease incidence. Cross-sectional studies may be the only feasible approach to diseases or disease states that do not necessarily come to medical attention, and might be difficult to study via a cohort or a case-control approach. For example, kidney dysfunction in workers exposed to heavy metals can be measured via the measurement of the excretion of small-molecular-weight proteins. Although the exact relationship of such excretion to subsequent renal disease is not known, it is possible that excretion of these proteins is an early marker of later symptomatic disease. It would not be possible to assemble "cases" of those excreting such proteins for a case-control study. A cohort study would be difficult because one would require a baseline measure of urinary protein followed by periodic urine samples, which involves many logistic difficulties. Another example might be serum-positivity for HIV infection in hospital workers exposed to blood products versus hospital workers not so exposed. Again, both case-control and cohort approaches would be either impossible or difficult.

There are three chapters on cross-sectional studies in Part III. The first chapter is a study of renal dysfunction among workers exposed to cadmium, the second is a study of carpal tunnel syndrome among workers in a grocery store, and the third is a study of cytogenetic changes in papaya workers exposed to a fumigant.

Chapter 8

Kidney Dysfunction in Cadmium Workers

MICHAEL THUN

In May 1985, workers at a cadmium production plant in Denver, Colorado, requested that the National Institute for Occupational Safety and Health (NIOSH) further evaluate health effects due to cadmium at their plant.

The plant had produced cadmium since 1925. Airborne exposures to cadmium dust and fume were extremely high in the past, but had decreased because of engineering controls and required use of respirators. The main function of the plant was to recover cadmium from "bag house" dust, a waste by-product of zinc smelters. Cadmium metal, oxide, and sulfide were sold for use in electroplating, pigments, plastics, nickel-cadmium batteries, and brazing. Small amounts of other metals (copper, selenium, thallium, arsenic, indium, and lead) had also been processed in localized areas of the plant, but the predominant exposure was to cadmium.

There had been several previous studies of health effects at the same facility, including three studies of kidney toxicity (NIOSH, 1977; Ellis et al., 1980; Smith et al., 1980a), one of pulmonary effects (Smith et al., 1976), and an ongoing retrospective cohort mortality study (Thun et al., 1985). The studies of kidney toxicity were cross-sectional studies that documented kidney dysfunction as measured by increased excretion of a small protein in the urine (beta-2-microglobulin), as well as altered calcium-phosphorus metabolism.

Chronic cadmium exposure causes a distinctive type of kidney disorder made manifest by increased urinary excretion of low-molecular-weight proteins, aminoacids, glucose, phosphate, and calcium. These abnormalities appear when cadmium reaches a certain critical concentration in the kidney. The kidney and the liver are the principal sites where cadmium is stored in the body. Some cadmium is eliminated from the body over time. However, the removal of cadmium occurs slowly, with a biological half-life of about 30 years.

A diagnosis of cadmium nephropathy among workers exposed to cadmium is usually made upon the observation of excessive excretion of small proteins such as beta-2-microglobulin (β-2-μg) and retinol binding protein (RBP). The excretion of these small proteins reflects damage to the proximal tubules of the kidney.

While the relation between cadmium and proximal tubular dysfunction is well known, the long-term effects of cadmium on other aspects of kidney function and health are less certain. One question involves whether cadmium workers experience an accelerated loss of glomerular function. Another involves adverse effects potentially related to disturbed calcium-phosphorus metabolism. Cadmium workers have an increased risk of kidney stones. Women exposed to cadmium in nonoccupational settings (through ingestion of cadmium-contaminated rice) developed painful bone fractures in an epidemic of so-called Itai Itai (Ouch Ouch) disease in Japan. Similar bone disease has occurred rarely in male cadmium workers.

Three issues needing clarification in 1985 concerned: (a) What is the dose-response relationship between cadmium exposure and kidney dysfunction as manifested by excessive excretion of β-2μg? (b) Does cadmium nephropathy progress to cause kidney problems besides proximal tubular dysfunction? (c) Is cadmium nephropathy reversible or does it persist or worsen after the cessation of exposure? All of these issues have regulatory significance, because they relate to the issue of whether the current occupational standard adequately protects workers from clinically important kidney dysfunction.

QUESTION 1. What epidemiologic study designs might be considered to assess kidney effects due to cadmium at the Denver plant? Consider as possible outcomes either tubular dysfunction or chronic renal disease. Discuss the advantages and disadvantages of different types of study design for each of these outcomes, in light of the issues needing clarification as outlined above.

Materials and Methods

The investigators decided to conduct a cross-sectional study of current and former workers. Objectives of the study were to assess dose-response relationships for several renal endpoints, to determine whether glomerular (as well as tubular) dysfunction was associated with cadmium, and to assess the persistence of nephropathy in former workers.

Because of temporary cutbacks at the plant, 26 of 45 (58%) workers listed on the union seniority roster had been laid off for at least six months. In considering who should be included in the target population for the cross-sectional study, investigators identified four potential groups; (a) 19 production workers still actively employed at the plant; (b) 26 workers who had been laid off in the preceding 6 to 7 months; (c) highly exposed, former workers identifiable from the retrospective cohort study who were still alive and might reside locally; and (d) an unexposed control group from the local area.

Investigators recruited 17/19 (89%) current production workers and 18/27 (67%) highly exposed former production workers who resided locally and were reachable by telephone. Two salaried workers and eight former short-term production workers not in the target population also were recruited after expressing interest in the study, although they were not part of the originally targeted groups. In addition, investigators enrolled 32 male workers from a local hospital who had never been occupationally exposed to cadmium. Nineteen of these hospital workers were employed in maintenance, shipping, and food service. Thirteen were office workers or professional staff.

QUESTION 2. What selection biases (differential participation due to exposure or illness) may have occurred in the recruitment? How could these be evaluated? (Assume that groups (a), (c), and (d) comprise the target population).

QUESTION 3. Why has a local control group been included in the study? How comparable are the hospital workers to the cadmium production workers?

The study included a questionnaire; measurement of height, weight, and blood pressure; and collection of "spot" daytime urine and serum samples. Questionnaire information included age and various medical conditions that cause kidney disease, such as diabetes, hypertension, and prostatic disease. Blood pressure was measured by a single examiner using a mechanical sphyngomanometer on the right arm of subjects who had been seated for at least 15 minutes. Measurements in urine included cadmium, beta-2-microglobulin, retinol binding protein, albumin, and three urinary enzymes. Measurements in serum included blood cadmium and serum creatinine. Laboratory specimens were processed immediately by a technician from the Centers for Disease Control reference laboratory who preserved and transported the samples.

At least four measures of cadmium exposure were potentially available for workers at the Colorado plant. Cadmium concentration in blood and/or urine could be measured at the time of a cross-sectional study. Blood cadmium is believed to reflect current exposure; urine cadmium reflects chronic exposure (although its relationship with cumulative exposure is not linear).

Length of employment in production areas of the plant provided a crude correlate of cumulative exposure. A fourth index of exposure had been derived in previous studies at this particular plant, by linking job histories with measurements of cadmium in the air of various departments over time. The cadmium air measurements were made routinely by the company. The raw data were subsequently refined by an industrial hygienist to estimate the cadmium actually inhaled by workers, adjusting for respirator usage and for changes in sampling methodology over time (Smith et al., 1980a; Smith et al., 1980b; Ellis et al., 1985). Respirators were judged to reduce cadmium exposure by 75%, based on surveys that measured cadmium inside and outside of respirators

TABLE 8.1 Estimates of Inhalation Exposures (mg/m³) by Plant Department and Time Period*

Department	Pre-1950	1950–54	1955–59	1960–64	1965–79	1980–85
Sampling	1.0	0.6	0.6	0.6	0.6	0.03
Roaster	1.0	0.6	0.6	0.6	0.6	—
Mixing	1.5	0.4	0.4	0.4	0.4	0.07
Calcine	1.5	1.5	1.5	0.4	0.15	0.4
Solution	0.8	0.8	0.4	0.4	0.04	0.04
Tankhouse†	0.04	0.04	0.04	0.02	0.02	0.04
Foundry	0.8	0.1	0.1	0.1	0.04	0.04
Retort	1.5	0.2	0.2	0.2	0.2	0.2
Pigment	0.2	0.2	0.04	0.04	0.04	0.08
Nonproduction†	0.09	0.05	0.04	0.024	0.02	0.007
Office & Lab	0.005	0.004	0.004	0.003	0.003	0.003
Non Plant‡	0.09	0.05	0.04	0.04	0.02	0.02
General Labor	1.166	0.485	0.485	0.331	0.279	0.041

*Original estimates from Smith (1976), with data on nonproduction and nonplant exposures added by Ellis (1980). Exposures from 1980–1985 added by NIOSH investigators based upon plant records and the assumptions of Smith (1976).

†Plant departments not directly involved in production of cadmium (maintenance in shop, laundry, litharge, indium, thallium, janitor, zinc, supervisory in plant, selenium).

‡Job classifications with reduced exposure conditions (guard, tailings dump, general labor outside plant).

worn by workers at this plant (Smith et al., 1980b). The estimate of inhaled cadmium in various departments over time are shown in Table 8.1.

QUESTION 4. Which measure of exposure would you expect to be most relevant to kidney toxicity and most appropriate to use in dose-response analyses?

Results

Full results may be found in Thun et al. (1989). Table 8.2 presents selected data for 32 unexposed hospital workers and 45 present and former cadmium workers. A categorical variable "exposed" is 0 for the hospital workers and 1 for the cadmium workers. Age (in years) was computed from birth date on the questionnaire. The variable representing external cumulative exposure is DOSE (in mg/m³-days). The variable B2PGC represents β-2-μg in urine (expressed as μg/g creatinine). This increases with proximal tubular dysfunction, and should be considered the outcome variable for cadmium-induced tubular proteinuria.

TABLE 8.2 Raw Data*

Exposed	Age (years)	Dose (mg/m³-d)	B2PGC (μg/g creat)	SBP (mm-Hg)	DBP (mm/Hg)	SCRE (mg/100 cc)
0	26.2	0.0	116.5	115	70	1.0
0	29.3	0.0	209.6	94	59	1.2
0	30.1	0.0	83.2	120	75	0.8
0	32.2	0.0	134.1	123	92	1.1
0	32.8	0.0	564.6	119	65	0.8
0	33.1	0.0	81.4	110	72	1.1
0	33.7	0.0	120.0	142	70	1.1
0	35.0	0.0	173.1	108	70	0.9
0	36.3	0.0	110.4	118	80	1.2
0	43.2	0.0	135.4	150	90	0.9
0	50.5	0.0	199.1	100	78	0.9
0	50.5	0.0	—	129	85	1.0
0	51.2	0.0	113.7	108	82	1.1
0	51.8	0.0	305.0	123	90	1.0
0	52.1	0.0	256.8	117	70	0.9
0	52.7	0.0	250.0	140	82	1.1
0	53.3	0.0	159.3	118	78	1.0
0	54.0	0.0	311.4	129	80	0.9
0	54.5	0.0	255.7	132	80	0.9
0	55.0	0.0	225.5	123	65	1.3
0	55.7	0.0	177.5	125	75	0.7
0	56.9	0.0	253.8	130	75	—
0	57.8	0.0	95.8	102	70	1.0
0	59.3	0.0	213.3	130	73	1.2
0	60.8	0.0	375.9	118	76	1.1
0	61.4	0.0	142.0	100	69	1.3
0	61.6	0.0	—	160	74	1.0
0	62.2	0.0	246.6	108	65	1.1
0	63.0	0.0	337.5	120	73	1.0
0	63.8	0.0	242.2	100	62	1.0
0	67.4	0.0	—	133	58	0.8
0	77.3	0.0	221.8	136	60	1.4
1	43.6	10.9	228.9	124	75	1.0
1	41.2	11.9	242.9	120	88	1.2
1	25.6	14.3	807.7	130	80	1.1
1	31.5	14.4	255.0	110	75	1.0
1	38.9	54.9	144.8	150	102	0.9
1	37.7	56.3	125.4	144	72	0.9
1	36.4	73.8	118.3	115	75	1.1
1	50.9	80.8	312.5	178	90	1.0
1	26.6	84.8	470.0	113	78	1.2
1	43.2	100.7	224.0	139	100	1.2
1	27.8	125.1	261.3	120	84	0.7
1	29.8	129.6	213.1	119	80	1.1
1	43.1	157.0	241.3	119	75	1.1
1	24.6	205.4	113.7	131	98	1.1
1	46.6	223.9	154.0	128	82	1.1
1	50.9	288.6	254.5	146	87	1.1

(*continued*)

TABLE 8.2 Raw Data (*Continued*)

Exposed	Age (years)	Dose (mg/m³-d)	B2PGC (μg/g creat)	SBP (mm-Hg)	DBP (mm/Hg)	SCRE (mg/100 cc)
1	60.9	299.3	150.0	131	79	0.9
1	70.7	299.8	596.9	133	72	1.0
1	57.7	312.9	1871	160	98	0.8
1	48.2	339.1	453.1	129	80	1.0
1	62.8	366.7	396.2	120	78	1.4
1	47.8	377.4	155.7	134	95	1.2
1	71.5	579.8	940.9	128	86	0.8
1	60.8	636.1	521.9	133	75	1.0
1	60.1	680.2	148.4	126	84	1.3
1	44.7	768.0	200.8	157	82	0.9
1	63.7	790.1	2803	158	92	1.4
1	70.7	791.4	891.7	138	85	0.9
1	66.6	957.6	10208	135	70	1.3
1	56.7	1033	2302	124	70	1.0
1	71.2	1041	122.0	157	89	1.4
1	50.6	1056	97.5	134	80	1.6
1	71.2	1150	328.1	152	74	1.4
1	69.8	1293	700.0	161	85	1.5
1	58.4	1953	488.0	111	64	1.3
1	65.4	1982	67632	154	71	2.6
1	64.4	2034	24288	175	90	2.5
1	77.5	2067	211.0	110	67	1.4
1	85.8	2179	512.5	108	65	1.1
1	63.1	2314	1144	136	73	1.0
1	65.8	2912	389.2	129	70	1.2
1	57.8	2957	172.8	154	85	0.9
1	65.1	3136	18836	128	80	1.4
1	73.7	5186	33679	143	70	1.8
1	65.4	5383	107143	129	75	1.4

*Course instructors may obtain these data on diskette from the author.

Systolic (SBP) and diastolic (DBP) blood pressure (in mm/HG) should be considered potential confounders, as should age. Serum creatinine (SCRE) (in mg/dl) increases as glomerular filtration rate decreases. It should be considered the outcome variable reflecting glomerular dysfunction.

QUESTION 5. How would you approach these data? (Note: Begin by considering data editing, transformation of certain variables, plotting, etc.)

QUESTION 6. How would you define an "abnormal" value of B2PGC in this population?

QUESTION 7. What statistical tests could be used to compare the cadmium workers as a group (EXPOSED = 1) to the hospital workers (EXPOSED = 0), ignoring any potential confounders?

QUESTION 8. Using the statistical tests identified above, determine whether the cadmium workers as a group have impaired renal tubular function (higher B2PGC) or reduced glomerular filtration rate (higher SCRE). (Note: Investigators used logs with base 10 when transforming data, and dichotomized B2PGC and SCRE into "normal" and "abnormal" using the following criteria: "High" β-2-μg = >486 μg/g creatinine, "high" serum creatinine $\geq$ 1.4 mg/100 dl).

QUESTION 9. How would you present your statistical findings comparing the exposed and unexposed workers?

QUESTION 10. How would you interpret the biological significance of these results?

The literature suggests that age may confound the relationship between cadmium and beta-2-microglobulin, since both cadmium exposure and β-2-μg excretion increase with age. Similarly, both age and blood pressure may confound the relationship between cadmium and serum creatinine. Questions 11–14 below require analyses using either linear or logistic regression with the data set attached for this exercise. These questions should be considered optional. Course instructors may obtain this data set, along with others, on diskette from the editor.

QUESTION 11. (Optional) Use linear regression to determine the relationship between cadmium dose and beta-2-microglobulin, controlling for age. How would you interpret the results? (In this analysis, use $\log_{10}$ B2PGC as the outcome variable, and DOSE as the exposure variable.)

QUESTION 12. (Optional) Use linear regression to determine whether blood pressure (systolic) confounds the relationship between cadmium and serum creatinine. The relationship between cadmium and serum creatinine is important, since this reflects whether or not cadmium causes an accelerated loss of overall kidney function. However, at least four scenarios are possible, as shown below: (a) represents the null hypothesis; (b) represents a direct causal relationship between cadmium and increased serum creatinine; (c) represents hypertension acting as a confounder, assuming cadmium dose and blood pressure are associated (by chance) in the data; and (d) represents hypertension acting as an intermediate between cadmium and increased creatinine. Which of these best fits the data?

(a) No association between cadmium and increased creatinine
(b) Cadmium→Kidney injury→Increased creatinine

(c) Hypertension→Kidney injury→Increased creatinine
Cadmium→Kidney injury→Increased creatinine
Cadmium↔Hypertension

(d) Cadmium→Hypertension→Kidney injury→Increased creatinine

Questions 13 and 14 concern logistic regression. Logistic regression can be used to determine the probability, or risk, of various types of kidney function being abnormal in relation to cumulative exposure to cadmium. The risk of normal versus abnormal kidney function in relation to cadmium exposure is more easily understood in individual and regulatory decision-making than is an equation resulting from linear regression, in which a continuous measurement of kidney function is predicted by level of cadmium exposure.

QUESTION 13. (Optional) Recall the criterium for defining "normal" and "abnormal" values of beta-2-microglobulin (abnormal is defined as the mean of the log transformed data plus two standard deviations). This criterium is based upon the small control group. How might outliers among the hospital workers influence the determination of risk?

QUESTION 14. (Optional) Using the same criteria for an elevated B2PGC (>=486 mg/g creatinine), determine the odds of abnormal B2PGC for exposed vs. unexposed. Also run a model with DOSE (a continuous variable, and then use the results from the model to determine the probability of abnormal B2PGC as a function of DOSE. Graph these probabilities (y-axis) versus DOSE.

Discussion

An important motivation for the study was to communicate meaningful results to workers, the union, and the company. Providing such information is usually a more central (and difficult) part of cross-sectional studies than it is for other epidemiologic study designs. One set of challenges involves notifying the individual workers (and often their physicians) about the meaning of their individual test results. A second challenge involves notifying the company, the union, and the scientific community about the meaning of the group results.

QUESTION 15. What issues often complicate the explanation of individual test results to workers and their physicians?

QUESTION 16. With respect to the company and union, how does one address the issues of whether workers with abnormal kidney function should be removed from further cadmium exposure?

When the present study was published (Thun et al., 1989), seven other published occupational studies had examined the prevalence of kidney dysfunction (tubular proteinuria) as related to cumulative exposure to airborne cadmium (Ellis et al., 1980; Thun et al., 1989; Falck et al., 1983; Kjellstrom et al., 1977; Jarup et al., 1988; Eliner et al., 1985; Mason et al., 1988). These studies vary somewhat in the criteria used to define tubular proteinuria, in size, and in the amount of exposure information available (see review, Thun et al., 1991). Nevertheless, the dose-response relationships can be compared among these studies. Figure 8.1 shows the prevalence of increased beta-2-microglobulin and retinol-binding protein excretion in relation to cumulative external exposure to cadmium based on these studies. Data from the present study (Thun et al., 1989) are shown as dark squares. Superimposed is a risk assessment model by the U.S. Occupational Safety and Health Administration (OSHA) (1990) based on the data of Ellis et al. (1980) and Falck et al. (1983). Also superimposed (dashed line) is a risk assessment from a metabolic model by Kjellstrom and Nordberg (1978).

Exposure to cadmium is expressed in two ways on the X-axis of Figure 8.1. The upper row refers to cumulative exposure in $\mu g/m^3$ (equivalent to DOSE $\times$ 2.74), and ranges from 0 to 18,000. The lower row refers to the permissible exposure limit (PEL), which would yield an equivalent cumulative exposure if experienced daily over a 45-year working lifetime. For example, a PEL of 1 $\mu g/m^3$ is equivalent to a cumulative 45-year exposure of $\mu g/m^3$-years (the cumulative exposure permitted by the U.S. official standard for cadmium dust (200 $\times$ $\mu g/m^3$-year) over 45 years).

QUESTION 17. Based on Figure 8.4 and the measurements shown in Table 8.1, are current exposures at this plant "safe"? (Note: The units in Table 8.1 are mg/m^3, whereas Figure 8.1 shows $\mu g/m^3$.)

QUESTION 18. What do you tell the workers and company when the legal standard is itself not protective?

This investigation served several useful purposes. From a service perspective, workers were informed of the results of their individual medical tests. From a research and public health perspective, the study provided additional information on the dose-response relationship between cadmium and various indices of kidney dysfunction and on the clinical significance of cadmium nephropathy. In particular, kidney dysfunction was found to involve both glomerular and a variety of tubular effects, which worsened with cadmium exposure. Regression analyses using a variable for time since last exposure showed that these effects persisted many years after cessation of exposure.

Since this study was completed, another study of cadmium workers found that kidney function (measured by serum creatinine) progressively worsened even after exposure had ceased (Roels et al., 1989).

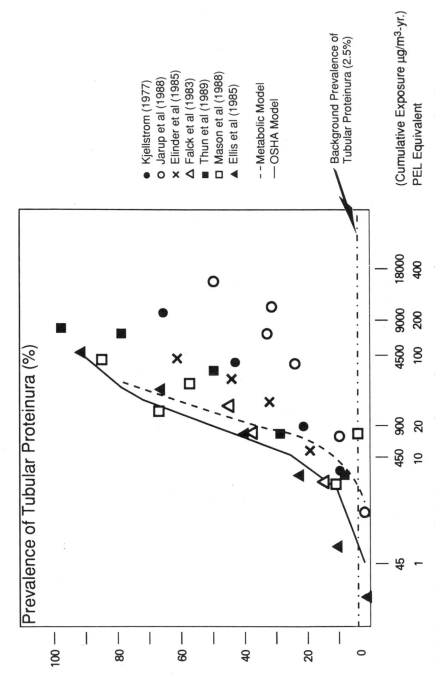

FIGURE 8.1 Prevalence of tubular proteinuria by cumulative exposure to cadmium in seven cross-sectional studies compared to prediction by the OSHA risk assessment and by the Kjellstrom metabolic model. Reprinted with permission of Am J Indust Med (from Thun et al., 1991).

This and other studies suggest a clear need for a more stringent occupational standard. However, the process of setting occupational standards in the United States is extremely slow, and at the time this exercise was written (June 1991) a new occupational standard for cadmium in the United States had not been officially established.

References

Ellis KJ, Cohn SH, Smith TJ: Cadmium inhalation exposure estimates: their significance with respect to kidney and liver cadmium burden. J Toxicol Environ Health 15:173–187, 1985.

Ellis KJ, Morgan WD, Zanai I, et al.: In vivo measurement of critical cadmium level in the human renal cortex. Am J Indust Med 1:339–348, 1980.

Elinder C, Edling C, Lindberg E, et al.: β-2-microglobulinuria among workers previously exposed to cadmium. Follow-up and dose-response analysis. Am J Indust Med 8:553–564, 1985.

Falck F, Fine L, Smith R, et al.: Occupational cadmium exposure and renal status. Am J Indust Med 4:541–549, 1983.

Jarup L, Elinder CG, Spang G: Cumulative blood-cadmium and tubular proteinuria: a dose-response relationship. Int Arch Occup Environ Health 60:223–229, 1988.

Kjellstrom T, Borin P, Rahnster B: Dose-response analysis of cadmium-induced tubular proteinuria. Environ Res 13:303–317, 1977.

Kjellstrom T, Nordberg G: A kinetic model of cadmium metabolism in the human being. Environ Res 16:248–269, 1978.

Mason H, Davison A, Wright A, et al.: Relations between liver cadmium, cumulative exposure, and renal function in cadmium alloy workers. Br J Indust Med 45:793–82, 1988.

NIOSH (National Institute for Occupational Safety and Health), Center for Disease Control, Public Health Service, HETAB Report #77-10, 1977.

OSHA, Occupational exposure to cadmium; proposed rule, Federal Register 29 CFR Part 1910:4052–4147, 1990.

Roels H, Lauwerys R, Buchet J, et al.: Health significance of cadmium-induced renal dysfunction: a five-years follow-up. Br J Indust Med 46:755–764, 1989.

Smith T, Anderson R, Reading J, et al.: Pulmonary effects on chronic exposure to airborne cadmium. Am Rev Resp Dis 114:161–169, 1976.

Smith T, Anderson R, Reading J: Chronic cadmium exposures associated with kidney function effects. Am J Indust Med 1:319–337, 1980a.

Smith T, Ferrell W, Verner M, et al.: Inhalation exposure of cadmium workers: effects of respirator usage. Am Indust Hyg Assoc J 41:624–629, 1980b.

Thun M, Elinder C, Friberg L: Scientific basis for an occupational standard for cadmium. Am J Indust Med 20:629–642, 1991.

Thun M, Osorio A, Schober S, et al.: Nephropathy in cadmium workers: assessment of risk from airborne occupational exposure to cadmium. Br J Indust Med 46:689–697, 1989.

Thun M, Schnorr T, Smith A, et al.: Mortality among a cohort of cadmium production workers—an update. JNCI 74:325–333, 1985.

ANSWERS

ANSWER 1a. Kidney dysfunction reflecting tubular damage. A cross-sectional study could advance beyond previous studies by attempting to relate various indices of kidney function, such as urinary β-2-μg, to quantitative estimates of cadmium exposure. Such a study has the advantage of providing further and stronger evidence that cadmium exposure is indeed the cause of the kidney dysfunction. Furthermore, quantitative dose-response relationships would be useful for regulatory purposes (setting an allowable exposure level). Cross-sectional studies are most appropriate for nonfatal, nondisabling (or slowly disabling) conditions that can be measured objectively. They play an important role in measuring changes in physiologic function as well as health outcomes. Markers of cadmium nephropathy (β-2-μg, RBP, etc.) are measurable, highly sensitive, and reasonably specific in working populations. Cadmium nephropathy (tubular dysfunction) develops slowly and seldom causes workers to leave employment.

While a cross-sectional study of urinary β-2-μg among current workers might be useful for the above reasons, it does not address the question of persistence of the dysfunction after exposure ceases, or the possible progression of the dysfunction to more serious kidney disease involving the glomerulus.

Persistence and progression would best be addressed by a longitudinal study in which the same individuals were followed over time with repeated measurements. Such a study would take several years and be very costly. Short of this, the issue of progression might be addressed cross-sectionally by measuring other markers of overall kidney dysfunction other than tubular effects. For example, serum creatinine provides a crude (insensitive) measure of loss of overall kidney function. If serum creatinine is increased, it suggests that clinically important loss of overall kidney function has occurred. Similarly, persistence can be addressed by including workers in the study who have not been exposed to cadmium for many years. Increased β-2-μg excretion among these workers would suggest relative irreversibility of tubular dysfunction.

ANSWER 1b. Increased incidence of chronic renal disease. A finding of increased chronic renal disease in this work force would indicate that the observed cadmium nephropathy had led to more serious kidney disease. A cross-sectional study of chronic renal disease would not be useful because men with chronic renal disease generally would be absent from the work force. The ongoing cohort mortality study might have detected an excess of chronic renal disease, but in general mortality studies are not very sensitive for renal disease, which is often not listed on death certificates. A population-based case-control study of end-stage renal disease (ESRD) might be possible if a list of incident ESRD patients over time could be obtained from a regional ESRD registry. However, such a study might have had little statistical power to detect an excess because the cadmium-exposed workers at the factory in question would form only a small part of the study population (the same problem would occur for a hospital-based case-control study). A case-control study of chronic renal disease within the company itself (nested within the cohort) might be useful, but the company had no record of who among its work force had developed chronic renal disease.

ANSWER 2. Selection biases pose an important problem in cross-sectional studies, since sick workers may have died, moved, or been unable to participate. Alternatively, workers who believe they have health effects due to exposure may be more or less likely to participate. The best safeguard against selection bias is having a well-defined target population and high participation rates. In this study, participation was good (89%) among current workers, but lower than desirable among former workers. One group that is of concern includes the ten "drop-in" workers who were not in the target population but participated in the testing. One should exclude these workers if their presence changed the results substantially. In this instance they were left in, since they increase the number of study subjects but have virtually no effect on dose-response coefficients.

ANSWER 3. In theory, a local nonexposed group is less necessary in dose-response analyses because more highly exposed workers can be compared to less exposed workers. However, in practice, a local nonexposed group was useful (a) to provide nonexposed referent values for specialized laboratory tests (which often vary greatly depending upon the techniques used to process and analyze specimens); and (b) to allow better control for age (which among the exposed group was correlated with both β-2-μg excretion, serum creatinine, and cumulative exposure to cadmium).

The professional and office workers at the hospital were not comparable to the exposed workers with respect to education and socioeconomic status. However, socioeconomic status was not an important potential confounder, because it was not thought to be strongly related to the outcomes of interest. Also, these workers were needed to provide a greater range in age than existed among the nonexposed maintenance workers. Age is an important potential confounder for the renal outcomes of interest.

ANSWER 4. The biologically relevant dose for kidney toxicity is the lifetime dose of cadmium taken up by the kidney; this dose is unknown for the workers in the study. A lifetime dose reflects cumulative (chronic) exposure rather than recent exposure. In this study, the estimate of cumulative external exposure may provide a better estimate of the biologically relevant dose than current urine cadmium concentration. First, urine cadmium among the currently exposed workers reflects not only cumulative absorbed dose but also excretion rates. Second, urine cadmium decreases after exposure ceases, whereas actual cumulative dose remains constant. Third, cumulative exposures based on air concentrations can be related directly to air concentrations in the workplace and to the question of the adequacy of current occupational standards.

(In practice, it was relatively easy to measure urine and blood cadmium to compare these to the estimate of cumulative external exposure. When this comparison was performed by the investigators, the estimate of external cumulative exposure was more closely associated with all of the health outcomes than were current blood and urine cadmium levels. Also, the estimates of cumulative external exposure were validated by comparing them to measurements of cadmium in kidney and liver (obtained by neutron activation) in selected workers at this plant (Ellis et al., 1985). There was a high correlation between the estimates of external exposure and the concentration of cadmium in kidney and liver.)

ANSWER 5. Useful strategies to assess the data include plots, checks for outliers or extreme values, and tests of normality (e.g., proc univariate in SAS). Skewed distributions can sometimes be "normalized" by log transformation. Both B2PGC and SCRE are distributed more normally after log transformation. Although normality is generally not a concern for t-tests in which each of the compared samples is of size 30 or greater, log transformation (to the base e or base 10) of B2PGC and SCRE is recommended in this exercise.

ANSWER 6. The criteria for "normal" and "abnormal" could be obtained from published referent data, or could be based upon the 97.5th (or 2.5th) percentile in a local control group. The problem with published normative data is that there may be substantial differences between laboratories, or the referent population may differ substantially in age or other important demographic characteristics from the study subjects. In this study, a value of 486.4 was chosen as the upper limit of "normal" for B2PGC, based upon the 97.5th percentile in the control workers (the mean of the log-transformed data plus two standard deviations).

ANSWER 7. Two statistical tests that could be used to compare the groups are Student's t-test (keeping B2PGC and SCRE as continuous variables), or chi-square (dichotomizing both B2PGC and SCRE into "normal" and "abnormal"). Comparisons between the groups are presented below.

ANSWER 8. The tables that follow show the results of Student's t-tests (comparing population means) and chi-square calculations (comparing proportions).

Comparison of Means Using Student's t-Test for Urinary beta-2-microglobulin and Serum Creatinine

Outcome	Cadmium (N = 45)		Hospital (N = 32)*		T-Statistic (d.f.)†	p-Value
	Mean	(SD)	Mean	(SD)		
Beta-2 (µg/g creatinine)						
Log 10 B2PGC†	611	(6.0)	189	(1.6)	3.45	.001
B2PGC**	6257	(19,364)	211	(103.9)	(72)	
Creatinine, serum (mg/dl)						
Log 10 SCRE‡	1.16	(1.30)	1.01	(1.17)	2.58	.011
SCRE**	1.20	(0.37)	1.03	(0.16)	(74)	

*Hospital workers N = 29 for B2PGC and N = 31 for SCRE.

†t-tests were conducted with the log-transformed data, which are more normally distributed. These t-tests are based on the assumption of equal variances in both groups (see formula in the Appendix), although a formal test for equal variances shows this assumption does not hold. A different t-test assuming unequal variances would be better for these data. The two tests yield similar results.

‡Values represent geometric mean and standard deviation. To obtain the mean of the logs (base 10), take the log of the geometric mean. To obtain the standard deviation of the logs, take the log of the standard deviation in the table. The mean of the logs and their standard deviation were used in the t-tests presented here.

**Values represent arithmetic mean and standard deviation.

Comparison of Proportions Using Chi-Square

	Cadmium Workers (N = 45)		Hospital Workers (N = 32)			
	(>486 µg/g creatinine)		(>1.4 mg/dl)		Chi-Square	p-Value
	#	%	#	%		
Beta-2-microglobulin, urine	18	40.0	1	3.5	12.35	<0.000
Creatinine, serum	12	26.7	1	3.2	7.11	0.008

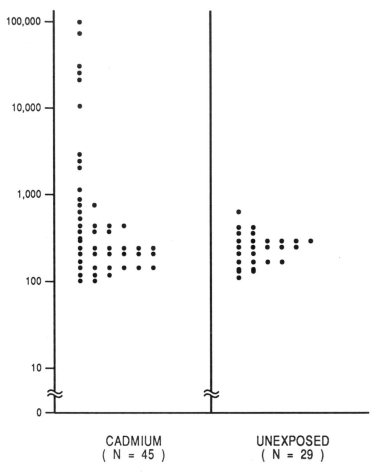

BETA-2-MICROGLOBULIN
(μg / g Creatinine in Urine)

CADMIUM
(N = 45)

UNEXPOSED
(N = 29)

FIGURE 8.2a Indices of renal function in the cadmium-exposed and unexposed workers. Reproduced with permission of Br J Indust Med (from Thun et al., 1989).

ANSWER 9. The results could be presented in tables as shown above. Both measures of central tendency (e.g., means or proportions) and the spread of the data (its variance) are important. Graphical presentation of the data with group means (Figure 8.2a and b) communicates a clear image of how the data are distributed. As illustrated by the figures, a subset of the cadmium workers have increased B2PGC and serum creatinine values, reflected in the higher group means.

ANSWER 10. Although the prognostic (biological) significance of increased urinary β-2-μg is not well established, the group data indicate that 40% of the cadmium workers have "tubular proteinuria." If present in

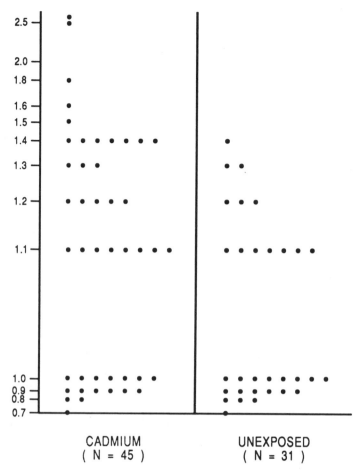

SERUM CREATININE
(mg / 100 cc)

FIGURE 8.2b Indices of renal function in the cadmium-exposed and unexposed workers. Reproduced with permission of Br J Indust Med (from Thun et al., 1989).

more than one measurement, this can be considered presumptive evidence of cadmium-induced renal tubular dysfunction. Serum creatinine values above 1.4 or 1.5 mg/100 cc generally reflect substantial loss of glomerular filtration rate, although because of the kidney's reserve, this may not cause clinical problems unless the loss in function progresses.

ANSWER 11. Stratified analyses and/or multivariate modeling could be used to identify and control for confounders. In this case, multiple linear regression provides the most efficient approach, given that the three variables of interest are all continuous. The table below shows the coefficient for cadmium (dose) in relation to beta-2-microglobulin ($\log_{10}$

B2PGC) with and without age (in years) in the model. The coefficient for cadmium decreases slightly when age is included in the model (suggesting that age is a weak confounder), even though age is not statistically significant. Figure 8.3 shows the data points, regression line, and 95% upper and lower confidence intervals for the model, including only the intercept and dose.

Regression Models for Beta-2-Microglobulin (expressed as Log_{10} B2PGC)

	β	S.E.	T	p	R^2 for Model
Intercept	2.323	—	—	—	0.50
Dose ($\times\ 10^{-4}$)	4.195	0.4976	8.43	<.0001	—
Intercept	2.108	—	—	—	0.50
Dose ($\times\ 10^{-4}$)	3.90	0.5729	6.80	0.0001	—
Age (years)	0.004	0.004	1.03	0.3	—

ANSWER 12. The regression models below show the association between cadmium alone, and cadmium-controlling for systolic blood pressure (SBP). As shown, the inclusion of SBP in the model causes only a small (8%) reduction in the coefficient for cadmium (indicating minimal confounding). This suggests that most of the association of cadmium with serum creatinine fits scenario (b). Were hypertension acting as an intermediate in the relationship, the inclusion of SBP in the model should cause the coefficient for cadmium dose to become much weaker and to lose significance. A model testing the association of SBP alone with SCRE yields a much smaller R^2 than that of cadmium alone. Thus, cadmium is a better predictor of SCRE than is blood pressure.

Regression Models for Serum Creatinine (expressed as Log_{10} SCRE)

	β	S.E.	T	p	R^2 for Model
Intercept	0.0139	—	—	—	0.23
Dose ($\times\ 10^{-4}$)	0.4384	0.0937	4.68	.0001	—
Intercept	−0.0747	—	—	—	0.24
Dose ($\times\ 10^{-4}$)	0.4125	0.0961	4.29	.0001	—
SBP	0.0007	0.0006	1.17	.25	—
Intercept	−0.1262	—	—	—	0.05
SBP	0.0013	0.0006	1.99	.05	—

ANSWER 13. Measurements of B2PGC are available for only 29 hospital workers. Of these, 28 had B2PGC levels below 376; the 29th had a B2PGC level of 564.6. Because of the small size of the control group, the single individual with the highest level has a major influence on the

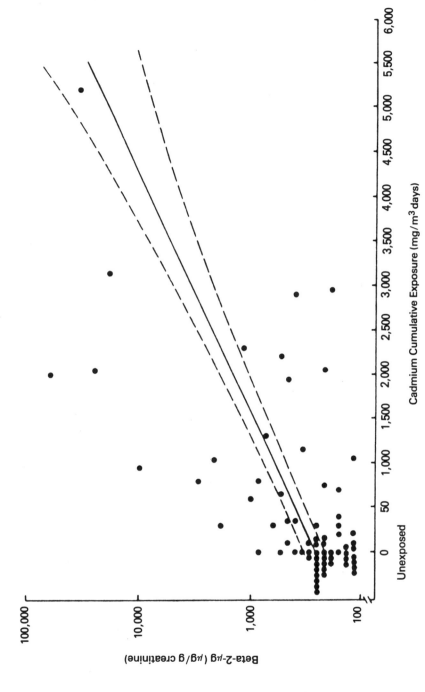

FIGURE 8.3 Regression of beta-2-microglobulin excretion versus cumulative external exposure to cadmium. Solid line indicates regression line. Dashed lines indicate upper and lower 95% confidence intervals. Reproduced with permission of Br J Indust Med (from Thun et al., 1989).

123

criteria for "abnormal." This may cause some underestimation of the proportion of "abnormal" workers at any exposure level. Nevertheless, the internal control group is preferable to any other source of referent values.

ANSWER 14. The odds ratio for abnormal beta-2-microglobulin, for an exposed versus nonexposed person, is 18.7 as determined by logistic regression (model with EXPOSED only). Age is significant in this model, but does not substantially confound the estimate for beta-2. Figure 8.4 shows the predicted probability (prevalence) of increased beta-2-micro-globulin in the urine in relation to dose. Figure 8.4 also shows the predicted probability of other renal abnormalities, showing patterns sim-ilar to that of B2PGC. The model indicates that the log odds or the log of $(p/1-p)$ equals $-1.9979 + .0013(DOSE)$. Most computer software pro-grams will solve for p (probability of abnormal beta-2), and also allow you to plot p versus DOSE.

ANSWER 15. Notifying individuals of their test results is often compli-cated by (a) experimental tests, the prognostic significance of which is not well understood; (b) unconventional collection procedures or units of standardization (e.g., the use of spot urine samples standardized per gram of creatinine, rather than per 24-hour collection); and (c) isolated "abnormal" values that may be due to laboratory error or variability within populations.

Each of these points could be discussed at length. In general, the most meaningful findings for patients and their physicians involve a pattern of multiple abnormalities relating to the same organ system or physiologic function. Isolated findings are difficult to interpret because of laboratory error or the variability that exists within populations.

ANSWER 16. Workers with clear-cut renal abnormalities (repeatedly in-creased beta-2-microglobulin and other evidence of renal tubular dys-function) should not have further exposure to cadmium. This decision should be based upon more than one measurement of beta-2-micro-globulin. If there are no unexposed jobs at the plant, or if changing jobs involves a reduction in pay, the union will need to negotiate with the company management to identify a fair assignment for the affected worker.

ANSWER 17. Exposures at this plant have equaled or exceeded 40 $\mu g/m^3$ in at least eight departments between 1980 and 1985. This would correspond to a cumulative exposure at or above 1,800 $\mu g/m^3$-years over 45 years, a level that is clearly not protective against renal tubular

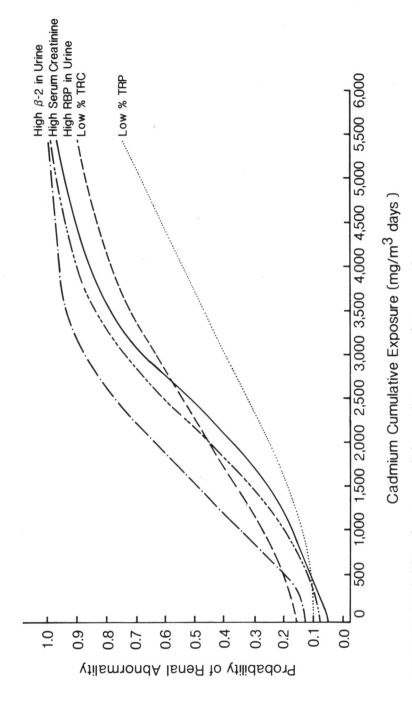

FIGURE 8.4 Probability of various renal abnormalities versus cadmium cumulative exposure. Abnormal renal tests defined as follows: High β-2-μg > 486 μg/g creatinine, high serum creatinine ≥ 1.4 mg/d1, high RBP > 321 μg/g creatinine, low tubular reabsorption of phosphate (TRP) < 69.4%, low tubular reabsorption of calcium (TRC) < 97.56%.

dysfunction. The current legal standard is even less protective, since it permits a cumulative exposure of 9,000 $\mu g/m^3$-years over 45 years.

ANSWER 18. The investigator has a responsibility to inform the workers and company when an official standard appears insufficiently protective. The company may respond in different ways to this information. Because occupational standards in the United States often lag behind scientific information, this is not an infrequent occurrence.

Chapter 9 | Carpal Tunnel Syndrome among Grocery Store Workers

ANA OSORIO

Carpal tunnel syndrome (CTS) involves entrapment of the median nerve in the region of the wrist and is associated with forceful and repetitive wrist motion. Studies of various occupational groups have demonstrated an increased prevalence of CTS: car seat sewers, aircraft engine assemblers, and butchers (Armstrong, 1979; Cannon, 1981; Falck, 1983).

CTS can present with one or more of the following symptoms and physical findings (Brain, 1947; Kendall, 1960; Phalen, 1972; Phalen, 1951):

1. Numbness, tingling, or burning pain on the palmar surface of the thumb, index, middle, and half of the ring finger (the median sensory nerve distribution of the hand)

2. Pain and tingling in this region, occurring mostly at night

3. Radiation or movement of the pain to the forearm and shoulder

4. Weakness of the thumb

5. Wasting of the muscle at the base of the thumb (thenar atrophy)

The nerve entrapment of CTS can be detected by measuring the velocity of an impulse traveling along the median nerve across the wrist. This examination is called a nerve conduction velocity (NCV) test of the sensory median nerve.

Mechanical factors that have been reported to be associated with CTS include the following (Armstrong, 1979; Cannon, 1981; Feldman, 1983; Smith, 1977; Tanzer, 1959; Tichauer, 1977):

1. Repeated wrist and finger flexion

2. Hyperextension of the wrist

3. Repetitive ulnar deviation

4. Pinching or grasping motions

5. Prolonged forceful use of the hands

6. Contact with vibratory tools or instruments

Several years ago, the California Department of Health and Human Services was asked to evaluate a reported cluster of CTS cases among employees at a large supermarket in the state. Nationwide, there are approximately 2.3 million persons employed in the grocery store industry (U.S. Dept. Labor, 1985).

QUESTION 1. What are the first steps in the evaluation of a potential occupational disease cluster?

In the preliminary investigation, four cases of CTS, all occurring among supermarket checkers, were confirmed based upon interviews with their respective personal physicians. There were 69 employees working at the store at the time of the study, of whom 15 were checkers. Supermarket checkers are employees who work at the checkout counter and pass grocery items across laser scanners.

QUESTION 2. Based on what you now know about CTS and the reported cluster of cases at the grocery store, would you conduct a further investigation of this problem? If so, why?

QUESTION 3. What type of study would be indicated at this point (please state the study null hypothesis, type of study design, and target population)?

Materials and Methods

It was decided to conduct an epidemiological investigation of this grocery store work force with the aim of assessing whether checkers or other employees with repetitive and forceful wrist-motion tasks experienced an increased prevalence of CTS, and, if there was a positive association, to recommend changes in the workstation or work habits that could decrease the risk of developing CTS.

The target population chosen included all current employees at the grocery store. In the actual study, retired employees were also studied, but the data for this case study will be restricted to current employees.

QUESTION 4. What would be the advantage of including ex-workers in the study?

A cross-sectional study design comparing those workers exposed to forceful and repetitive wrist motions with those workers with no such exposure required the development of an exposure classification scheme and a case definition for CTS.

The exposure classification scheme was derived by an ergonomist and an industrial hygienist during various observational visits to the grocery store. They conducted visual inspections of employees at work and noted those job tasks that required the kind of high-risk hand movements associated with CTS. Each job was assigned to a high-, medium-, and low-risk category based on the type of work tasks required and the average amount of time spent performing these tasks per week (Table 9.1). In the study itself, the prevalence of CTS among workers in the high-exposure category (including checkers, meat cutters, and cake decorators) was to be compared to the prevalence among workers in the two categories with relatively less exposure.

QUESTION 5. There are more systematic methods to classify study subjects into exposure groups, according to risk of CTS. Can you think of what these might be?

The prevalence of CTS among the three exposure categories was assessed by medical interview, physical examination, nerve conduction velocity testing, and vibratory machine examination of the median nerve. For the purposes of this exercise, only the results of the medical interview and nerve conduction tests will be discussed.

The interview consisted of a questionnaire administered in-person or by telephone, which included questions about pertinent medical and job factors. The nerve conduction test measured the velocity of nerve impulses in the sensory median nerve of both wrists, in meters per second (M/sec). Slowing of the

TABLE 9.1 Exposure Classification Scheme
for Grocery Store Workers*

Risk Category	Job Task
High	Bakery, applying icing on cakes
	Butcher
	Grocery checking
Medium	Bagger
	Bakery, all tasks except cake icing
	Pricing
	Shelf stocking
Low	Flower shop attendant
	Office work
	Produce work
	Stockroom work

*The assignment of study subjects into the high-, medium-, and low-risk categories also included an assessment of whether the person performed the stated work task 20 or more hours per week. Those persons conducting high- or medium-risk tasks less than 20 hours per week were assigned the next-lower category.

TABLE 9.2 Two Case Definitions

CTS by symptom history
Pain, tingling and/or numbness on the palm side of the first three fingers and
   half of the fourth finger (median nerve area)
Onset or exacerbation since working on the current job

CTS by median nerve conduction velocity abnormality
Sensory median nerve conduction velocity of 44 M/sec or less*

---

*This value is used as a cutoff point by the reference laboratory from which the portable
electrodiagnostic equipment was borrowed.

conduction velocity would indicate an abnormal median nerve function, consistent with the diagnosis of CTS.

All of the interview and testing procedures were standardized and performed
by trained personnel who were unaware of the exposure classification of each
participant. There were two case definitions (see Table 9.2) used for CTS,
partly because it was expected that not everyone would consent to the nerve
conduction velocity test (this test requires a momentary, minute electrical shock
to the wrist).

Results

For a full description of the results, see Osorio et al. (1992).

Fifty-six of 69 grocery store workers (81%) participated in the study by
completing the interview and medical exam. For the nerve conduction velocity
test, the participation rate was 32/69 (46%). The distribution of various demographic traits such as race, gender, and age for the participant group differed
little from the distribution of these traits for the nonparticipants.

QUESTION 6. Using the data presented at the end of this exercise (Table
9.4), fill in the values for Table 9.3 (NOTE: the actual data have been
slightly altered for the purposes of this exercise.) Course instructors may
also obtain these data on diskette from the editor. Conduct chi-square
significance tests to determine whether the percentage of males and
females differs by exposure category, and whether a positive medical
history differs by exposure category. Based on these tests, are these sex
and medical history factors possible confounders for the exposure-
disease analysis?

QUESTION 6a. As an optional exercise, conduct an analysis of variance
(ANOVA) to test for differences in mean age or alcohol-years between the
three exposure categories (continuous variables). Might these variables
act as confounders?

TABLE 9.3 Demographic and Medical Data by Exposure Group

	Exposure Group			
	Low	Medium	High	All
No. of subjects				
Mean age (std. dev.)	( )	( )	( )	( )
No. of women (column %)*	( )	( )	( )	( )
No. of men (column %)	( )	( )	( )	( )
Mean alc-yrs† (std. dev.)	( )	( )	( )	( )
No. with high-risk medical history‡ (column %)	( )	( )	( )	( )
No. w/out high-risk medical history (column %)	( )	( )	( )	( )

*% of the column (exposure category) total for sex or medical history.

†Alc-yrs = (average # drinks/month) × (total # years drinking).

‡Indicates potentially high-risk medical history (current estrogen or birth-control medication, diabetes, pregnancy, thyroid disease, rheumatoid arthritis, or past hand surgery).

For the definition of a CTS case based on the medical history (either or both wrists affected), the following number of cases were identified for the three exposure groups:

> Low exposure = 0 cases/10 subjects surveyed
> Medium exposure = 3 cases/30 subjects
> High exposure = 10 cases/16 subjects

The overall prevalence of a history indicative of CTS among the employees was 23%.

QUESTION 7. Calculate the prevalence risk ratio and the chi-square test of association (and associated p-value), comparing the prevalence of history-based CTS in the high-exposure group with the prevalence of the combined medium/low-exposure group. Comment on why the two lower-exposure groups were combined and suggest alternative analyses.

For the CTS definition based on median nerve conduction (either or both wrists affected), the following number of cases were identified in each exposure group:

Low exposure = 0 cases/5 subjects surveyed
Medium exposure = 1 case/15 subjects
High exposure = 4 cases/12 subjects

An overall prevalence of 16% was obtained for the occurrence of an abnormal median nerve velocity among the study subjects.

QUESTION 8. Calculate the prevalence risk ratio comparing the prevalence of CTS (definition based on nerve conduction velocity) in the high-exposure group with the prevalence of the combined medium/low-exposure group. Calculate the chi-square test of significance and the corresponding p-value.

QUESTION 9. Is there an apparent dose-response for CTS by exposure category, using either definition of CTS? Calculate the Mantel-extension tests for positive trends (dose response) between (1) CTS by history and exposure, and (2) CTS by NCV and exposure. Use as scores 1 for low exposure, 2 for medium exposure, and 3 for high exposure.

To evaluate the median nerve conduction velocity (NCV) results as continuous variables, the mean values across the exposure categories were calculated. The NCV data were calculated for each wrist separately. Checkers and other workers in the high-exposure group used both wrists during the course of their jobs, and may have worsened the nerve function of either wrist.

QUESTION 10. Using the data in the Appendix, fill in the following table. Is there an apparent dose response for nerve conduction for either wrist? As an optional question, conduct an ANOVA to determine if there are any significant differences between exposure groups for either wrist.

| | Exposure Group (score) | | | |
	Low (1)	Medium (2)	High (3)	All
No. of subjects				
Mean median nerve velocity, right wrist				
Mean median nerve velocity, left wrist				

QUESTION 11. As an optional exercise, use linear regression to test whether there are significant linear trends between NCV (for each wrist separately) and the predictor variables of "yrswork" (total years worked at grocery store). Determine whether age or sex need to be included in the model. Examine the coefficient for years worked when the data set is restricted to the 12 people in high-exposure jobs, versus when the data set is restricted to the 20 people in low- and middle-exposure jobs. Interpret the results. Write down the equation for the model that predicts NCV as a function of years worked for those in high-exposure jobs.

Discussion

The high-exposure group had significantly higher CTS prevalence than other grocery store workers in this study. Dose-response relationships were seen between the three exposure groups and the outcome variables of CTS symptoms and abnormal median nerve conduction velocity. Results were consistent for either case definition of CTS. These results nevertheless need to be treated with caution due to relatively small sample size, particularly for the nerve conduction results.

The medical and epidemiological literature contains numerous studies that demonstrate an association between CTS and certain types of hand and wrist motion. Although the literature for grocery store workers is not extensive, the association between CTS and meat cutters is well established (Falck, 1983; Armstrong, 1982; Viikari-Juntura, 1983). Regarding checkers specifically, the literature contains some inconclusive studies but does provide some indication that hand symptoms (and possibly CTS) are a major problem (Barnhart, 1987; Rosenstock, 1985; Margolis, 1987; Morgenstern, 1991). The ergonomic literature identifies various workstation-design problems encountered in this work force and describes some primary preventive measures that are thought to decrease the risk of acquiring CTS (Wallersteiner, 1986).

The possibility that symptomatic employees have already left the work force cannot be ruled out. This situation would tend to strengthen any association that was found in the relatively healthier survivor population. Eighty-one percent of the work force completed the questionnaire portion of the evaluation.

Potential confounders for CTS and abnormal nerve conduction were identified prior to the study onset and based on an extensive review of the medical literature. However, the possibility that a potential confounder was not recognized cannot be ruled out.

Observational bias was minimized by the use of standardized case definitions, exposure categories, interviews, and testing protocols. All examiners were blinded as to the medical and occupational history of each subject.

In summary, the employees in this grocery store perform job tasks that require varying degrees of forceful and repetitive motions, and they appear to be at increased risk for CTS. This is especially true of the checkers, meat cutters, and cake decorators. The types of jobs in supermarkets fall into common

TABLE 9.4 Data for CTS Study*

ID	RISKCTS	YRSWORK	AGE	ISEX	ALCYR	IMEDHX	VELR	VELL	CTSCASE
01	1.00	3.00	21.74	.00	.00	.00	48.28	53.85	0.00
02	2.00	5.00	23.11	.00	4.00	.00	50.00	53.85	0.00
03	2.00	6.00	50.12	1.00	.00	1.00	51.85	46.67	1.00
04	2.00	7.00	24.11	1.00	18.00	1.00	56.00	61.85	0.00
05	3.00	.80	25.39	1.00	24.00	1.00	50.00	61.85	0.00
06	2.00	6.00	42.89	1.00	10.00	.00	58.33	58.33	1.00
07	3.00	3.00	27.74	1.00	18.00	1.00	58.33	53.85	0.00
08	2.00	1.00	31.89	1.00	81.00	.00	—	—	0.00
09	3.00	3.00	20.90	.00	.00	1.00	50.00	53.85	0.00
10	2.00	.30	26.17	.00	30.00	.00	51.85	53.85	0.00
11	1.00	4.00	41.48	.00	40.00	.00	56.00	60.87	0.00
12	2.00	1.00	38.46	1.00	70.00	.00	53.85	51.85	0.00
13	3.00	7.00	31.45	1.00	1.00	1.00	48.28	50.00	1.00
14	1.00	1.00	18.52	1.00	2.00	1.00	53.85	56.00	0.00
15	3.00	7.00	25.24	1.00	48.00	1.00	50.00	50.00	1.00
16	2.00	1.00	19.19	1.00	10.00	.00	53.85	53.85	0.00
17	3.00	5.00	36.53	1.00	.00	.00	58.33	63.64	1.00
18	3.00	9.00	53.03	1.00	64.00	1.00	38.89	42.42	1.00
19	2.00	7.00	59.24	1.00	.00	.00	40.00	48.28	1.00
20	3.00	2.00	45.59	1.00	25.00	.00	53.85	58.33	0.00
21	3.00	7.00	62.59	1.00	.00	.00	37.84	35.90	0.00
22	3.00	9.00	37.94	.00	195.00	.00	38.89	36.84	1.00
23	1.00	.80	18.58	.00	15.20	.00	45.16	46.67	0.00
24	2.00	1.00	18.86	.00	44.00	.00	50.00	53.85	0.00
25	2.00	1.00	22.22	.00	93.00	.00	56.00	58.33	0.00
26	2.00	1.00	39.14	1.00	.00	1.00	53.85	56.00	0.00
27	1.00	2.00	17.81	1.00	11.00	.00	53.85	58.33	0.00
28	2.00	8.00	28.23	.00	50.00	.00	56.00	56.00	0.00
29	3.00	2.00	46.20	1.00	40.00	1.00	53.85	53.85	0.00
30	2.00	3.00	20.46	.00	18.00	.00	53.85	51.85	0.00
31	2.00	1.00	33.84	1.00	5.00	.00	53.85	56.00	0.00
32	3.00	7.00	24.10	1.00	.00	1.00	43.75	53.85	1.00
33	2.00	6.00	28.18	.00	396.00	.00	—	—	0.00
34	1.00	.80	27.96	.00	30.00	.00	—	—	0.00
35	3.00	7.00	48.76	.00	.00	1.00	—	—	1.00
36	2.00	7.00	36.51	1.00	150.00	.00	—	—	0.00
37	2.00	1.00	19.55	1.00	.00	.00	—	—	0.00
38	2.00	.80	18.77	.00	50.00	.00	—	—	0.00
39	2.00	.80	19.27	.00	6.00	.00	—	—	0.00
40	1.00	1.00	22.99	1.00	2.00	.00	—	—	0.00
41	2.00	.30	19.64	1.00	24.00	.00	—	—	0.00
42	2.00	7.00	29.53	1.00	40.00	.00	—	—	0.00
43	2.00	7.00	26.98	1.00	10.00	1.00	—	—	0.00
44	3.00	12.00	29.19	.00	72.00	.00	—	—	1.00
45	2.00	.30	21.06	.00	6.00	.00	—	—	0.00
46	2.00	.50	23.63	.00	.00	.00	—	—	0.00
47	2.00	.50	24.16	1.00	.00	.00	—	—	0.00
48	2.00	.90	18.51	1.00	.80	.00	—	—	0.00
49	1.00	.50	18.73	.00	.00	.00	—	—	0.00
50	2.00	2.70	22.05	.00	.00	.00	—	—	0.00

(continued)

TABLE 9.4 Data for CTS Study* (*Continued*)

ID	RISKCTS	YRSWORK	AGE	ISEX	ALCYR	IMEDHX	VELR	VELL	CTSCASE
51	2.00	9.00	27.34	1.00	48.00	.00	—	—	0.00
52	3.00	.90	21.17	1.00	4.00	.00	—	—	1.00
53	1.00	4.00	30.70	1.00	6.00	1.00	—	—	0.00
54	2.00	1.00	21.74	1.00	2.00	.00	60.87	56.00	0.00
55	3.00	2.00	23.30	1.00	20.00	1.00	—	—	1.00
56	1.00	2.00	19.75	.00	48.00	.00	—	—	0.00

Number of cases listed = 56

Definitions of variables:

RISKCTS = low- (1.0), medium- (2.0), and high- (3.0) risk exposure category. These values can be used as "scores" for the exposure categories.

YRSWORK = years subject has worked at the study grocery store.

AGE = age in years.

ISEX = sex of subject, male (0.0) or female (1.0).

ALCYR = alcohol years = (average number of alcohol units/month) × (total years with this pattern). An alcohol unit is defined as one can or bottle of beer, or one glass of wine, or one shot of hard liquor.

IMEDHX = potentially high-risk medical history (current estrogen or birth control medication, diabetes, pregnancy, thyroid disease, rheumatoid arthritis, or past hand surgery) is present (1.0) or absent (0.0).

VELR = sensory median nerve conduction velocity of the right wrist, M/sec.

VELL = sensory median nerve conduction velocity of the left wrist, M/sec.

CTSCASE = CTS case based on medical history is 1.0, a noncase is 0.0.

*The values presented here differ slightly from those used in the actual data analysis presented in Osorio et al. (1992).

patterns, with similar exposures to cumulative hand and upper-extremity trauma. The basic principles of good ergonomic design can be used to prevent or diminish the risk of musculoskeletal injury.

References

Armstrong TJ, Chaffin D: Carpal tunnel syndrome and selected personal attributes. JOM 21(7):481–486, 1979.

Armstrong TJ, Foulke JA, Joseph BS, et al.: Investigation of cumulative trauma disorders in poultry processing plant. Am Indust Hyg Assoc J 43:103–116, 1982.

Barnhart S, Rosenstock L: CTS in grocery checkers: cluster of work-related illness. West J Med 147:37–40, 1987.

Brain WR, Wright AD, Wilkson M: Spontaneous compression of both median nerves in the carpal tunnel. Lancet 1:277–282, 1947.

Cannon LJ, Bernacki EJ, Walter SD: Personal and occupational factors associated with carpal tunnel syndrome. JOM 23(4):255–258, 1981.

Falck B, Aarnio P: Left-sided carpal tunnel syndrome in butchers. Scand J Work Environ Health 9:291–297, 1983.

Feldman RG, Goldman R, Keyserling WM: Peripheral nerve entrapment syndromes and ergonomic factors. Am J Indust Med 4:661–681, 1983.

Kendall D: Etiology, diagnosis, and treatment of paraesthesia in the hands. Med J 2:1633–1640, 1960.

Margolis W, Kraus JF: Prevalence of carpal tunnel syndrome in female supermarket checkers. JOM 29:953–956, 1987.

Morgenstern H, Kelsh M, Kraus J: A cross-sectional study of hand/wrist symptoms in female grocery checkers. Am J Indust Med 20:209–218, 1991.

Osorio AM, Ames R, Jones J, et al.: Carpal tunnel syndrome among grocery store workers: a medical and neurodiagnostic cross-sectional study. Submitted for publication, 1992.

Phalen G: Carpal tunnel syndrome. Clin Orthop 83:29–40, 1972.

Phalen G: Spontaneous compression of median nerve at the wrist. JAMA 145(15): 1128–1133, 1951.

Rosenstock L, Barnhart S, Longstreth W, et al.: CTS in Seattle grocery workers. Health Hazard Evaluation NIOSH, August 1985.

Smith E: Carpal tunnel syndrome: contribution of flexor tendons. Arch Phys Med Rehab 58:379–385, 1977.

Tanzer RD: Carpal tunnel syndrome. J Bone Joint Surg 41A(4):626–634, 1959.

Tichauer E, Gage H: Ergonomic principles basic to hand tool design. Am Indust Hyg Assoc J 38:622–634, 1977.

U.S. Department of Labor, Annual Report, Washington D.C., 1985.

Viikari-Juntura E: Neck and upper limb disorders among slaughterhouse workers. Scand J Work Environ Health 9:283–290, 1983.

ANSWERS

ANSWER 1. The initial steps in the evaluation of a potential occupational disease cluster are similar to that of a nonoccupational cluster:

1. Formulation of a case definition for the disease or medical condition of interest (e.g., CTS).

2. Confirmation of the diagnoses of the index cases (e.g., meeting CTS criteria as defined by step 1).

Should the confirmed cases plausibly result from occupational risk factors, and should the prevalence of the cases initially appear to be excessive compared to what one might expect, investigators may wish to proceed to evaluate the cluster with a formal study. A formal study would involve identification of all cases in the work force, calculation of disease incidence or prevalence rates, and determination if the incidence or prevalence among the exposed population was greater than expected.

ANSWER 2. The preliminary investigation revealed four true cases of CTS; other types of neuromuscular injury of the hand or wrist were excluded. There is no general population rate for CTS that is available, but a preliminary prevalence rate of 26.7% (4/15) among checkers appears to be more than one might expect. A comparison group was needed to assess whether a true statistical cluster existed.

Checkers constitute a potentially high-risk occupational group because all of the mechanical risk factors, apart from the vibratory exposure, may be present in the tasks required of them. Other grocery store workers may also work in jobs with these risk factors as well. It is already known that other occupations requiring high-risk wrist motions have shown an association with CTS. Furthermore, there are many grocery store workers nationwide that could also be at risk for CTS. Based on the initial apparent cluster, biological plausibility, and the size of the population at risk, further study is warranted.

ANSWER 3. (a) One possible study null hypothesis is that there is no difference between the prevalence of CTS among checkers versus other grocery store workers with no exposure to repetitive wrist movement in their jobs. Another possible null hypothesis would be that there is no difference between the prevalence of CTS among all workers with jobs involving high-risk wrist motions at the store (checkers and any others), when compared to the remaining workers.

(b) The study design would be a cross-sectional type.

(c) The target population for the study would be all the employees at this grocery store.

ANSWER 4. The researcher would be able to detect the CTS cases that left work because of their disability. The current work force is in essence a survivor population that is healthy enough to perform their job. The absence of ill workers from the current work force is a problem typical of many cross-sectional studies of disease that are potentially debilitating.

ANSWER 5. The method to classify exposure groups here relied on a visual inspection of tasks and ranking them according to observed high-risk hand and wrist motions associated with CTS, conducted by an ergonomist. An ergonomist is a specialist who evaluates the adequacy of the workstation, tools, machines, and job tasks for a given worker. A visual inspection of the worker performing his/her job tasks is a preliminary evaluation. Because of poor cooperation from the management of the grocery store under study, the study ergonomist was unable to conduct a more detailed job analysis. A more detailed analysis would have consisted of videotaping each job sequence and concurrent electromyography to estimate the required force associated with each job task. Nonetheless, the exposure classification scheme used here should have been adequate to divide the work force into meaningful exposure groups for comparison. One example of a more detailed exposure assessment of checkers can be found in Harber et al. (1992).

ANSWER 6 and 6a. Chi-square tests show that medical history, but not sex, differs significantly across exposure categories. Note that due to the small sample size (see accompanying table) some of the expected numbers used in calculating the chi-square are less than 5, so that the chi-square test may be somewhat inaccurate. Nevertheless, the test indicates that medical history could confound the analysis of CTS by exposure, if it were also associated with CTS. Age is also a potential confounder since the ANOVA shows that the mean age differs by exposure category (higher-exposure categories are older), and age is often associated with health outcome of any type. Alcohol-years does not differ significantly across exposure categories, and would not be expected to act as a confounder.

Demographic and Medical Data by Exposure Category

| | Exposure Group | | | | | |
| | Low | Medium | High | All | | |
No. of subjects	10	30	16	56	p-value	Type of Analysis
Mean age (std. dev.)	23.8 (7.6)	27.8 (10.0)	34.9 (12.8)	29.1 (11.1)	0.03	ANOVA (F-test)
No. of women (column %)	4 (40)	18 (60)	12 (75)	34 (61)	0.20	Chi-square (2 degrees of freedom)
No. of men (column %)	6 (60)	12 (40)	4 (25)	22 (39)		
Mean alc-yrs* (std. dev.)	15.4 (17.7)	25.5 (24.7)	25.7 (30.1)	23.7 (62.0)	0.59	ANOVA (F-test)
No. with high-risk history† (column %)	2 (20)	4 (13)	10 (63)	16 (29)	p = .002	Chi-square (2 degrees of freedom)‡
No. w/out high risk history	8 (80)	26 (87)	6 (37)	40 (71)		

*Alc-yrs = (average # drinks/month) × (total no. years drinking)

†Indicates potentially high-risk medical history (current estrogen or birth-control medication, diabetes, pregnancy, thyroid disease, rheumatoid arthritis, or past hand surgery).

‡Note that the expected in one of the nine cells of this 3 × 2 table is less than 5, so that the chi-square test may be invalid.

ANSWER 7. An unadjusted prevalence risk ratio of 8.33 for a history of CTS-like symptoms between the highest and lower two exposure groups was obtained. This risk ratio was statistically significant, judging by the chi-square test of association (19.0, p < .001). Again, the chi-square test here is somewhat suspect due to the fact that one of the cells has an expected value of less than 5. Fisher's exact test, used in such a case, also showed the association to be highly significant.

Logistic regression controlling for potential confounders (age, medical history) yielded similar results.

		History-based CTS		
		Present	Not present	
Exposure group:	High	10	6	16
	Low/medium	3	37	40
		13	43	56

Combining the two lower exposure groups enabled the calculation of a single measure of risk for one group versus another. It would also be theoretically possible to calculate two separate risk ratios (high versus low, medium versus low), with the purpose of assessing a dose-response trend (higher risk with higher exposure). However, the fact that there are no cases in the low-exposure group makes it impossible to calculate these risk ratios (although some investigators arbitrarily add 0.5 to the empty cell to overcome this problem). A dose-response trend may still be calculated even in the presence of empty cells, via the Mantel-extension test.

ANSWER 8. A prevalence ratio of 6.67 was obtained in the comparison of nerve conduction–based CTS between the high- and medium/low exposure groups. The chi-square test of association was 4.57, which (with one degree of freedom) yields a p-value of 0.03. Again, the chi-square test is somewhat suspect here because two of the cells have expected values less than 5.0. The Fisher's exact test (two-tail) for association yields a p-value of 0.053. Control of confounders (age, medical history) via logistic regression yielded odds ratios that fell just short of conventional statistical significance ($p < 0.05$), but that continued to show an increased risk of poor nerve conduction velocity for the highly exposed compared to those with less exposure.

		CTS as based on median nerve conduction velocity		
		Present	Not present	
Exposure group:	High	4	8	12
	Low/medium	1	19	20
		5	27	32

ANSWER 9. An apparent dose-response relationship resulted when the prevalence of CTS-like symptoms was compared across the exposure categories. A similar dose-response relationship was seen for the prevalence of an abnormal median nerve conduction velocity, although the prevalences are smaller than that of the respective history-based CTS prevalences.

The Mantel trend test yields a chi-square of 16.1 (p-value < 0.001) for prevalence based on history, and a chi-square of 4.01 (p-value = 0.045) for prevalence based on NCV. These results show that the apparent trend observed in the data was statistically significant.

ANSWER 10.

| | Exposure Group | | | |
	Low	Medium	High	All
No. of subjects	5	15	12	32
Mean median nerve velocity, right wrist	51.43	53.34	48.50	51.23
Mean median nerve velocity, left wrist	55.14	53.77	50.36	52.71

For either wrist, the high-exposure group has a lower mean than the low- or medium-exposure groups. However, a test via an ANOVA shows that the three exposure groups do not differ significantly (for either wrist). The data do appear consistent with a downward trend in NCV with more exposure, especially with the left wrist.

ANSWER 11. Regression results using "years worked" as the exposure variable are shown below. There was a statistically significant correlation between the median nerve conduction velocity for each wrist and the total years worked at the study grocery store. Age and sex did not significantly predict NCV after the inclusion of years worked. The negative correlation with velocity suggests that increasing exposure produces a decrease of the median nerve conduction velocity. The correlation between years worked and decreasing NCV was significant for the high-exposure group, but not for the combined low/medium exposure group.

Results were the same for both wrists. For either wrist, the regression line for the high-exposure subjects has a slope of about −1.8, which suggests that each year worked in a high-exposure job would result in a 1.8 M/sec decrease in the nerve velocity.

These results indicate a dose-response with duration for the high-exposure group only. These results must be interpreted with caution because of the small sample size. Nonparametric correlation coefficients generally parallel the parametric results.

Regression line: $Y = C + BX$

Y	X	B (se)	C	P Value (B)	R-Square
All subjects					
(n = 32)					
VELR	YRSWORK	−1.02 (.34)	55.12	0.005	0.23
VELL	YRSWORK	−1.02 (.34)	56.59	0.005	0.23
High exposure					
(n = 12)					
VELR	YRSWORK	−1.82 (.55)	57.9	0.008	0.53
VELL	YRSWORK	−1.79 (.70)	59.6	0.03	0.39
Low/med exposure					
(n = 20)					
VELR	YRSWORK	−0.16 (.42)	53.3	0.71	0.01
VELL	YRSWORK	−0.25 (.34)	59.6	0.48	0.03

References for Answers

Harber P, Bloswick D, Peña L, et al. The ergonomic challenge of repetitive motion with varying ergonomic streses. J Occup Med 34: 518–528, 1992.

Chapter 10

Cytogenetic Study
of Workers Exposed
to Ethylene Dibromide

KYLE STEENLAND

Ethylene dibromide (EDB) is a colorless gas that has been widely used until recently as a pesticide to fumigate grain, treat soil, and fumigate fruit. EDB has been shown to be highly mutagenic, and carcinogenic at multiple sites in animals. Two mortality studies have been conducted among small cohorts of chemical workers exposed to EDB, but there have been inconclusive regarding cancer due to very small sample sizes and uncertainty regarding the actual exposures of the workers (Ter Haar, 1980; Ott et al., 1980). EDB has also been shown to have toxic effects on sperm in animals.

In the years 1983 to 1984 there was great public concern about the cancer risk posed by EDB, which had been found in trace amounts in cereals sold in supermarkets and also in groundwater (due to its use as a soil fumigant). Both the Environmental Protection Agency (EPA) and the Occupational Safety and Health Administration (OSHA) were considering regulatory action that would restrict the use of EDB and lower permissible exposure limits for workers. At the time OSHA standard for worker exposure was 20 parts per million (ppm). In late 1983, OSHA began regulatory procedures aimed at lowering that standard to 100 parts per billion (ppb) (0.1 ppm). In 1982 investigators at the National Institute for Occupational Safety and Health (NIOSH) sought to develop more information about the health effects of EDB, particularly regarding cancer. Further information was needed quickly, given the public concern and the imminent regulatory processes.

There were relatively few workers exposed to EDB, and these were distributed among many sites. They included workers in chemical plants either manufacturing or using EDB, agricultural workers applying EDB for soil fumigation, and workers applying EDB for fumigation of grain or fruits.

QUESTION 1. Is there any study design that might answer the question about whether EDB caused cancer in humans? What other outcomes besides cancer might be worthwhile to study?

Materials and Methods

NIOSH investigators chose to conduct a cross-sectional study of workers exposed to EDB during the fumigation of papaya to kill fruit fly larvae. A group of nonexposed referent workers would also be studied. Investigators chose to study cytogenetic outcomes (chromosomal aberrations (CAs) and sister-chromatid exchanges (SCEs)) and reproductive outcomes (damage to sperm), with data on both outcomes to be collected from the same workers at the same time. The focus of this exercise is the cytogenetic study. The reproductive study (Ratcliffe et al., 1987) will not be considered further here.

CAs result from mutations in the DNA, which in turn cause chromosomes to show breaks and rearrangements when viewed under a microscope during metaphase at mitosis (after the lymphocytes have been cultured and stimulated to divide) (see Figure 10.1). SCEs are not mutations, but instead are the exchange of genetic material between a pair of sister chromatids during mitosis, thought to be part of a normal process of DNA repair (see Figure 10.2). Most known human carcinogens cause CAs or SCEs in human lymphocytes. While EDB had not been tested for CAs or SCEs in human lymphocytes, tests in Chinese hamster cells had been positive for both CAs and SCEs.

The cytogenetic outcomes were to be measured in the peripheral lymphocytes of workers and referents, after drawing a venous blood sample. The blood sample would be taken to a lab, so that the lymphocytes could be cultured and stimulated to divide. Following standard procedures, cell division would be halted after one or two cycles, cells would be stained, and cells in the metaphase of mitosis would be identified. CAs would be counted in 200 cells (metaphases) for each study participant, while SCEs would be counted in 80 cells (metaphases) per person. The total number of CAs per person, and the average number of SCEs per cell (or per chromosome) for each person, would then be calculated. In turn, these numbers would be averaged across the entire exposed group and this overall average compared to the corresponding figure for the referents. Background rates for CAs are about 1 per 200 cells, while SCEs are much more common, averaging about 8 per cell. Age, sex, and smoking are either known or suspected to affect the number of CAs and SCEs (the association between SCEs and smoking is the strongest). Lymphocytes live anywhere from a few months to 20 years. Cytogenetic damage occurring far in the past could in theory be observed, but in practice such early damage appears to be repaired or else the affected cells die, so that in general it is recent exposure that causes observed cytogenetic alterations. For this reason, recent estimates of exposure are the most relevant ones.

QUESTION 2. Prior to beginning a study of cytogenetic changes in the target population, what other data need to be obtained?

QUESTION 3. At this "design stage," prior to data collection, what strategies should be adopted to control for the suspected confounding effects of smoking, age, and sex?

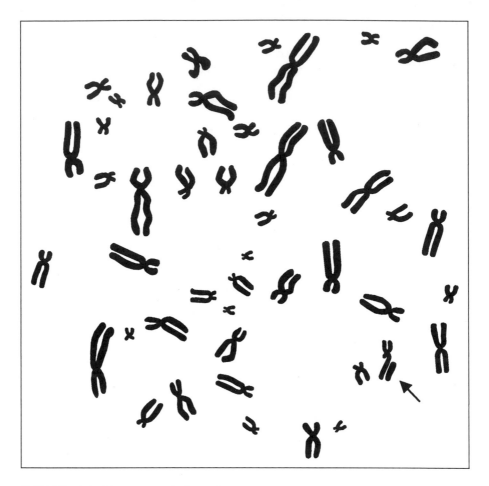

FIGURE 10.1 Chromosomal aberration.

QUESTION 4. What practical problem might one expect at this initial stage of the study? What would be the first steps to be taken?

QUESTION 5. What type(s) of data analysis might be expected once the data had been collected?

Employers of six papaya packing plants in Hawaii were contacted. Papaya in Hawaii was fumigated with EDB prior to export. The plants received the fruit, washed it, fumigated it, and packed it for export. The packing plants were small, often employing a dozen or fewer workers. The owners of the plants were cooperative. Many of them worked at the plant and were also potentially exposed. Workers at one plant were unionized, and the union was also contacted. The first step was to conduct an industrial-hygiene survey, characteriz-

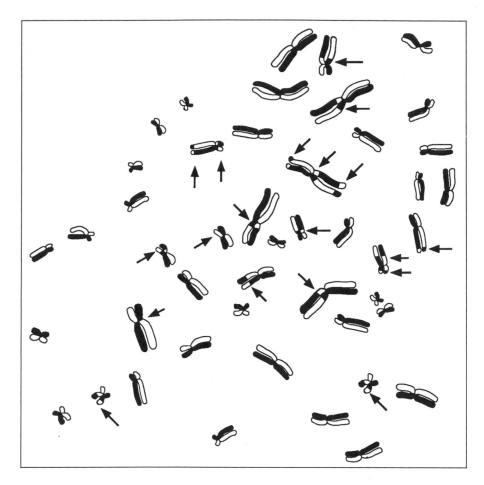

FIGURE 10.2 Sister-chromatid exchange.

ing exposure at the six plants. Full-shift personal samples (n = 82) were collected in late 1982 and early 1983. These samples were collected prior to the identification of the actual study subjects, although they were conducted at the six targeted plants.

Management and union at a nearby sugarcane plant were also contacted, and their participation solicited. Management was cooperative and the sugarcane workers interested. The sugar plant workers operated a mill that produced sugar from the cane. They were offered $40 for participation. The exposed workers were not offered any money for their participation, under the assumption that they would have a direct benefit from the study in that potential genetic or reproductive damage due to EDB exposure would be discovered.

Most workers were male, and the study was restricted to men. Sixty exposed workers agreed to participate, and 40 nonexposed sugar plant workers.

QUESTION 6. Discuss the potential advantages of using sugarcane workers as referents, compared to other possible sources. What other groups might have been used?

QUESTION 7. Full cytogenetic analyses cost about $200 per person. Given this expense, should the study include all those who agreed to participate, or could meaningful results be obtained with fewer people? What kind of calculations could be done prior to initiating the study to determine needed sample size?

Investigators from a laboratory in California collaborated with NIOSH for the cytogenetic analysis. Five millimeters of blood were to be drawn for each study participant and flown to California within 24 hours of collection.

Results

A full description of study results can be found in Steenland et al. (1986). Here, for the sake of brevity, only the SCE results are discussed.

The industrial-hygiene survey confirmed that the papaya plant workers were exposed. Their levels averaged about 100 ppm, which was the new standard proposed by OSHA. The study would yield information about effects on workers exposed to EDB at the proposed standard, and such information would be particularly relevant.

Table 10.1 shows exposure levels across all six plants by the three principal job categories (statistical analyses showed no significant differences between plants).

Everyone who worked in the plants was exposed. The relative number of samples reflected the relative numbers of workers in the job categories. Sorters and packers were the most common jobs. Forklift operation was more specialized. Forklift drivers entered the fumigation chambers to load and unload the fruit, and had somewhat higher exposures than sorters and packers.

TABLE 10.1 Average EDB Exposure Levels by Job, Based on Full-Shift Personnel Samples

Job	EDB in ppb (number of samples)
Sorter/packer	68 (n = 63)
Forklift operator	96 (n = 17)
Fumigator	116 (n = 2)

TABLE 10.2 Descriptive Data on Study Participants

	Exposed (n = 60)	Nonexposed (n = 40)
Mean age	35	30
Percentage cigarette smokers	48	38
Packs per day, smokers	1.1	0.9
Percentage marijuana smokers	40	23
Percentage white	13	20
Percentage Philipino	30	48
Percentage Japanese	17	15
Percentage Hawaiian/mixed Asian	40	17
Cups of coffee/day	1.8	1.9
Drinks per week	13.4	8.2

Fumigation usually was not a specific job, but instead was done by a variety of plant personnel. Often it consisted of little more than turning a valve to allow the gas to enter the chamber. At only one plant was there a specific person assigned to fumigation.

The samples were not collected from the same workers who eventually participated in the study, although there was some overlap. In the analysis of cytogenetic outcomes, it was not possible to use sampling data actually collected on each exposed worker. In any case, the relevant exposures presumably were not the current ones but rather exposures that had occurred at some point in the recent past.

No industrial-hygiene samples were collected among the referent workers, who were not exposed to EDB. Work history data were collected from them, however, to discover any past employment in the packing plants (past EDB exposure), as well as any exposure to other toxins in the sugar mill.

Table 10.2 shows the demographic data for both exposed and referent participants.

There was some imbalance in the age and smoking characteristics of the two groups, which would possibly be of importance in the analysis. Marijuana smoking was surprisingly prevalent, and might also be a factor in the analysis (marijuana smoking was freely admitted, and appeared to have little or no social stigma attached). Racial characteristics differed somewhat as well. Coffee consumption was similar. Alcohol consumption was actually rather similar, although one extremely heavy drinker among the exposed skewed the distribution.

QUESTION 8. Why would the fact that there was "some imbalance" in the smoking distribution between exposed and referents have some possible importance in the analysis? What is the definition of a confounder?

TABLE 10.3 Average SCEs by Exposure and Cigarette Smoking

	Exposed to EDB (std. err. mean)	Not Exposed (std. err. mean)
Smokers	0.2078 (.0052)(n = 29)	0.2008 (.0068)(n = 15)
Nonsmokers	0.1732 (.0033)(n = 31)	0.1731 (.0039)(n = 25)

Results for SCEs are shown in Table 10.3. In the table the SCEs have been calculated per chromosome (there are 46 chromosomes per cell) rather than per cell.

QUESTION 9. Upon inspection, do these data indicate any exposure effect for EDB? Is smoking an effect modifier (define)? Do these data indicate an effect of cigarette smoking on SCEs? Calculate a test for the difference between the two means, and consult a table to obtain the associated (two-sided) p-value, for exposed smokers versus referent smokers. Interpret the meaning of the p-value. Is this test significant at the traditional 0.05 alpha level? What analyses might be conducted next?

Further analyses for EDB exposure compared (1) those with more than five years duration of exposure (the average) to those with less than five years exposure, (2) those who reported dermal exposure or who reported smelling EDB to those who did not, and (3) forklift drivers/fumigators to sorters and packers. None of these comparisons showed any significant differences, and stratification for smoking did not change the negative results.

Simple comparisons of means did not show any hint of an EDB effect, but did indicate that cigarette smoking increased SCEs. An unexpected finding was that marijuana smoking increased SCEs among those who did not smoke cigarettes, as shown in Table 10.4.

QUESTION 10. How would you interpret these data? Conduct a t-test to compare the means between marijuana smokers and marijuana non-smokers among those who do not smoke cigarettes. Are these means significantly different? What further analyses might be done to provide even stronger evidence of a true association between cigarette smoking and SCEs, or between marijuana smoking and SCEs?

A regression analysis was conducted in which SCE level was the dependent variable, and a variety of predictor variables (e.g., X rays, viral infections, alcohol consumption, cigarette smoking, marijuana smoking, age, race, prescription medicine) were included in the model along with EDB exposure.

One of the simpler models included the predictor variables EDB exposure (0/1),

TABLE 10.4 Mean SCEs by Smoking Status

	Marijuana Smokers (std. err. mean)(n)	Nonusers of Marijuana (std. err. mean)(n)
Cigarette smokers	0.2097 (.0067)(n = 15)	0.2039 (.0056)(n = 27)
Non–cigarette smokers	0.1860 (.0048)(n = 17)	0.1669 (.0025)(n = 37)

cigarette smoking (0/1), marijuana smoking (0/1), and age (continuous). Analyses were also run in which the quantity of cigarettes per day was considered, as well as the frequency of smoking marijuana. The purpose of these last analyses was to test for a dose-response for cigarettes and marijuana use and SCEs.

QUESTION 11. The data for analyses described above are shown in Table 10.5 (course instructors may obtain these data on diskette from the author). As an optional exercise, enter these data into a computer and conduct the regression with exposure ("exp"), cigarette smoking ("cig") and marijuana smoking ("marj") dichotomized, and age ("age") as a continuous variable (note that the variable "marj" is missing for four individuals). Determine which of the four predictor variables is a significant predictor of SCEs. Determine whether the residuals for the full model with the four variables are distributed normally. How would you test an interaction or effect modification between marijuana use and EDB exposure (i.e., suppose the effect of EDB was seen only in those who smoked marijuana)?

Consider a simple model with just cigarette smoking (0/1) and marijuana smoking (0/1). Since both variables are dichotomous, this is an analysis of variance. How do you interpret the R-square for the model as a whole? Is the interaction term between cigarette smoking and marijuana smoking significant, as you might deduce from Table 10.4?

Now use continuous variables ("cigpks" and "marjinwk") for the amount of cigarettes smoked and the frequency of marijuana smoking. Do these analyses suggest a dose-response for cigarettes and SCEs? For marijuana and SCEs?

Discussion

EDB exposure, at these relatively low levels, was not associated with SCEs in these data (nor with CAs). This study had a relatively large sample size, and had relatively good power to detect an increase in SCEs. Hence, the results are somewhat reassuring in that exposure at the levels being proposed by OSHA at the time (and subsequently enacted) had no cytogenetic effects.

TABLE 10.5 EDB Study Data

SCE	Age	Cigpks	Cig	Marj	Exp	Marijnwk
0.1646	32	0.0	0	0	0	0
0.1867	29	0.5	1	1	0	7
0.1693	33	0.0	0	0	0	0
0.1870	21	0.0	0	1	0	2
0.1781	28	0.0	0	0	0	0
0.1643	40	0.0	0	0	0	0
0.1736	24	0.0	0	0	0	0
0.2228	31	1.0	1	0	0	0
0.2221	39	1.0	1	0	0	0
0.1921	28	1.0	1	1	0	1
0.1586	23	0.0	0	1	0	1
0.1931	42	0.0	0	—	0	—
0.1668	29	0.0	0	—	0	—
0.2273	41	1.0	1	1	0	7
0.2280	27	0.0	0	1	0	2
0.2112	35	1.0	1	0	0	0
0.1726	51	0.0	0	0	0	0
0.1683	36	0.0	0	0	0	0
0.1969	29	0.0	0	0	0	0
0.1455	36	0.0	0	0	0	0
0.2617	30	1.0	1	0	0	0
0.2098	56	0.0	0	1	0	1
0.1995	32	1.0	1	0	0	0
0.1616	29	0.5	1	0	0	0
0.1466	33	0.0	0	0	0	0
0.1587	61	0.0	0	0	0	0
0.1754	30	1.0	1	1	0	2
0.1999	35	1.0	1	0	0	0
0.1711	35	1.0	1	0	0	0
0.2062	24	1.0	1	0	0	0
0.1517	28	0.0	0	0	0	0
0.1820	57	0.0	0	0	0	0
0.1771	20	0.0	0	1	0	7
0.1544	28	0.0	0	0	0	0
0.1706	43	0.0	0	0	0	0
0.2053	25	0.5	1	0	0	0
0.1889	27	0.0	0	0	0	0
0.1583	60	0.0	0	0	0	0
0.1691	42	1.0	1	0	0	0
0.1627	40	0.0	0	0	0	0
0.2278	32	2.0	1	1	1	1
0.1571	19	0.0	0	0	1	0
0.2215	24	1.0	1	1	1	1
0.1554	19	0.0	0	0	1	0
0.1672	59	0.0	0	0	1	0
0.2474	29	2.0	1	1	1	2
0.1816	20	0.0	0	1	1	1
0.2030	34	1.0	1	0	1	0
0.1495	30	0.0	0	0	1	0
0.2039	19	1.0	1	0	1	0

(*continued*)

TABLE 10.5 EDB Study Data (*Continued*)

SCE	Age	Cigpks	Cig	Marj	Exp	Marijnwk
0.2055	23	0.5	1	1	1	7
0.1806	21	0.0	0	1	1	2
0.1858	23	0.0	0	0	1	0
0.1892	25	1.0	1	1	1	7
0.1845	35	0.0	0	0	1	0
0.1606	23	0.0	0	0	1	0
0.1801	19	0.0	0	1	1	5
0.1917	35	0.5	1	1	1	1
0.2078	40	1.0	1	0	1	0
0.1633	60	0.0	0	0	1	0
0.1691	23	0.0	0	1·	1	3
0.1856	24	1.0	1	1	1	7
0.2163	30	0.5	1	0	1	0
0.1679	18	0.0	0	0	1	0
0.1981	58	0.0	0	0	1	0
0.2526	24	1.0	1	1	1	7
0.1603	43	0.0	0	0	1	0
0.1869	33	0.0	0	1	1	3
0.2100	30	1.0	1	0	1	0
0.1677	24	0.0	0	0	1	0
0.2379	58	1.0	1	0	1	0
0.1672	23	0.0	0	0	1	0
0.2079	22	0.0	0	1	1	7
0.1637	52	0.0	0	1	1	1
0.1775	19	0.0	0	1	1	1
0.2156	32	1.0	1	0	1	0
0.2461	26	0.5	1	1	1	1
0.1990	26	0.0	0	1	1	2
0.1616	26	0.0	0	1	1	2
0.1937	20	0.0	0	0	1	0
0.2621	38	2.0	1	0	1	0
0.1859	26	0.5	1	1	1	7
0.2102	28	1.0	1	1	1	7
0.1825	41	2.0	1	—	1	—
0.2058	42	1.0	1	—	1	—
0.2328	35	1.0	1	0	1	0
0.1978	39	1.0	1	0	1	0
0.2142	20	0.0	0	1	1	3
0.1712	25	0.0	0	0	1	0
0.1983	47	1.0	1	0	1	0
0.1591	22	0.0	0	0	1	0
0.2131	32	2.0	1	0	1	0
0.1421	32	1.0	1	0	1	0
0.1747	22	0.0	0	0	1	0
0.1624	27	0.0	0	0	1	0
0.1379	28	1.0	1	0	1	0
0.1230	30	0.0	0	0	1	0
0.1798	20	0.0	0	1	1	7
0.1942	20	1.0	1	0	1	0
0.2014	25	2.0	1	0	1	0

*Course instructors may obtain these data on diskette from the editor.

The well-known association between SCEs and cigarette smoking was observed, and showed a dose-response. Findings were similar for marijuana smoking, although the effect was observed only in nonsmokers of cigarettes, and was weaker than the effects of cigarette smoking.

References

Ott M, Scharnweber H, Langner R: Mortality experience of 161 employees exposed to EDB. Br J Indust Med 37:163–168, 1980.

Ratcliffe J, Schrader S, Steenland K, et al.: Semen quality in papaya workers with long-term exposure to EDB. Br J Indust Med 44:317–326, 1987.

Steenland K, Carrano A, Ratcliffe J, et al.: A cytogenetic study of papaya workers exposed to ethylene dibromide. Mutat Res 170:151–160, 1986.

Ter Haar G: An investigation of possible sterility and health effects from exposure to EDB. Banbury Report 5:167–188, 1980.

ANSWER 1. A retrospective cohort study of workers exposed to EDB in the past, using cancer mortality or incidence as the outcome, would be the most typical study design for answering the cancer question. However, this approach was not feasible for several reasons. Most exposed cohorts were small, causing the potential cohort study to have little power to detect a cancer risk. Furthermore, many worksites in which EDB was used had little or no historical information to identify workers exposed in the past, with the exception of the chemical industry. Chemical workers who were exposed were often few in number and had little exposure, because many chemical processes were enclosed and involved little EDB exposure. Chemical workers also had been exposed to many other toxic chemicals, making interpretation of a possible positive cancer result more difficult. Finally, even if a cohort study were possible, it would take several years to assemble a cohort and do the necessary follow-up.

A population-based case-control study of cancer incidence for certain cancer outcomes was not possible either. Animal studies showed cancers at many sites, and it was not clear what particular sites were of primary interest in humans. Furthermore, while much of the general population would be exposed to trace amounts of EDB, such exposure would be quite difficult to measure. Substantial (occupational) exposure to EDB would be very rare. In this situation, a population-based or hospital-based case-control study would have little power to find an EDB-related cancer excess.

As an alternative, it was decided to study cytogenetic outcomes—chromosomal aberrations (CAs) and sister-chromatid exchange (SCE). An elevation of these outcomes above background would indicate that EDB was having a direct effect on the genome, which in turn *might* indicate an increased risk of cancer. Both outcomes are usually measured in peripheral lymphocytes, easily obtained from a small venous blood sample.

The decision to study cytogenetic outcomes was made because it was not possible to directly study cancer among EDB workers. An elevation of cytogenetic changes in the exposed workers would be an indication that exposure was affecting the genes, and would raise concern, although no inference could be made about subsequent cancer risk.

ANSWER 2. Industrial-hygiene sampling data were needed to confirm that the papaya workers had appreciable exposure to EDB, and to determine the relative levels of exposures among different job categories. Some workers at the papaya packing plants, for example, might not have had any exposures, while others might have had high exposures.

ANSWER 3. Data on smoking, age, and sex could be collected and control over these variables exercised at the analysis stage, or the exposed and referent groups could be matched on these variables prior to data collection. Matching could be pair-matching or frequency-matching. In the latter, a set of exposed workers of a certain age, sex, and smoking type would be matched to a set, of equal size, of referents with the same distribution of age, sex, and smoking variables. Matching would typically be done in a study such as this one only if the exposed group was quite small, so that it would be difficult to control confounding at the analysis stage.

Another possibility is that the study could be restricted to those of a specific age, sex, or smoking habit. For example, the study might be restricted to males if there were very few exposed females.

ANSWER 4. Cross-sectional field studies require the cooperation of those to be studied. In this case it would be necessary to contact the papaya workers and see if they would agree to have a blood sample taken (not to mention the sperm sample). This contact, unless the workers were unionized and could be approached directly, would require identifying employers and soliciting their cooperation, in order to contact the workers. Cooperation of both workers and management would also be required for any industrial-hygiene sampling of EDB exposures. Finally, a group of nonexposed referents would have to be identified and their cooperation sought as well. A practical difficulty is that employers might not believe the study was in their interest and might not cooperate. Exposed workers might not be worried about EDB and might be unwilling to donate blood or sperm. Referents might see no reason whatsoever to participate. One question is whether either exposed or referent groups would be paid for their cooperation.

ANSWER 5. A simple univariate t-test comparing the mean number of CAs or SCEs in each group would probably be the first step in the analysis. If pair-matching were used to control for the effects of confounders, a t-test for paired data could be used. If no matching was used for control for the effects of age, smoking, and sex, these factors could be incorporated into the analysis by using linear regression in which the outcome was the number of CAs or SCEs and the independent variables includes exposure, age, sex, and smoking. Typically, the exposure variable might be dichotomous (i.e., yes or no). It might also be possible to use a continuous variable for exposure, such as estimated cumulative dose. The use of such a continuous variable, however, would require assigning a specific quantified exposure level to each participant in the study. This, in turn, would require either gathering industrial-hygiene data on the exposure of each subject, or perhaps using industrial-hygiene data to assign a level to each job in the packing plant and then assigning that exposure level to any worker in that job.

ANSWER 6. There are many potentially confounding factors in a cytogenetic study, beyond the suspected factors of age, sex, and smoking. The study of cytogenetic outcomes is fairly recent, and hence factors influencing these outcomes are not well understood. Therefore, it was desirable to find a group of referents who were similar to the exposed population regarding socioeconomic status, diet, etc. For this reason, a group of workers from the same area, but not exposed to EDB, would be a good source. Another possibility would be members of the same community as the exposed workers, recruited possibly through neighborhood organizations (e.g., churches, clinics). The sugar plant workers were convenient in that they were all at one worksite and could be recruited with minimal difficulty. An unmatched group was selected, and confounders were controlled at the analysis stage. The sample size was large enough so that such control could be exercised in the analysis.

ANSWER 7. Typically, before the study is begun, an investigator will calculate the sample size needed to detect a certain level of difference between the exposed and referents (with a specified power). The formula for such calculations using categorical data to be analyzed in contingency tables is presented in the Appendix. Similar calculations can be done for data to be analyzed via a difference in means (e.g., t-test). In this case, investigators approached all workers in all six papaya plants and the sugar mill workers to see who would volunteer. Sixty exposed and 40 referents did so. Investigators then calculated that with this sample size the study had 80% power to detect a 15% increase in SCEs (exposed versus referent), and a 45% increase in CAs, using an alpha level of 0.05.

This power was felt to be adequate. The investigators decided to test everyone who had volunteered.

ANSWER 8. One definition of a confounder is that it is a variable that is associated both with exposure and outcome, and hence can distort the observed relationship between these two. SCEs are known to be increased by smoking. The fact that the exposed and referent groups differed somewhat on smoking implies that smoking might confound the analysis of the association between EDB and SCEs. Age was another potential confounder, in that exposed and referent groups differed somewhat in age and increased age had been associated with increased SCEs in some reports. Race, marijuana, and alcohol consumption were also potential confounders because they differed between exposed and referents, but unlike age and smoking there had been no reports in the literature indicating that these variables were associated with SCEs.

ANSWER 9. There appears to be little or no difference between the exposed and referent group, for either smokers or nonsmokers. Smoking does not modify the effect of EDB, in that the lack of an exposure effect is seen for both smokers and nonsmokers. A t-test between exposed and referent smokers yields a t-statistic of 0.80 with an associated (two-sided) p-value of 0.43. The p-value represents the probability that a difference between the groups as big as or bigger than the one observed would have occurred by chance, if in fact no difference existed (the null hypothesis). Taking $p = .05$ as the cutpoint for significance, EDB has no significant association with SCEs for smokers (the same result is obtained for nonsmokers). Cigarette smoking itself, however, is associated with a highly significant elevation of SCEs. Further analyses might adjust for other potential confounders in a regression, or examine subgroups among the exposed. Such subgroups might include those with longest exposure, or those in job categories with presumably higher exposure.

ANSWER 10. Cigarette smokers have higher SCEs than those who don't smoke cigarettes, regardless of marijuana use. Those who use marijuana show higher SCE levels than those who do not use marijuana, but only among those who don't smoke cigarettes. A t-test among nonsmokers of cigarettes shows that the mean SCE is significantly higher among marijuana smokers ($t_{52} = 3.90$, $p = .0003$). It is likely that the strong effect of cigarettes overwhelms the effect of marijuana use among cigarette smokers. Marijuana consumption is frequently limited to a few marijuana cigarettes a day or less, while cigarette consumption usually is higher, around 20 cigarettes per day (one pack). In these data, cigarette smoking is acting as an effect modifier in evaluating the relationship between marijuana smoking and SCEs. Further analyses for these variables might test for a dose-response, by determining if those who smoked more heavily (either cigarettes or marijuana) showed the highest SCE levels.

ANSWER 11. Neither EDB exposure nor age is a significant predictor of SCEs, but both cigarette smoking and marijuana smoking are. Age has a positive coefficient, indicating some SCE increase with age, as predicted by the literature. It is possible that the relative narrow age range in this study population made the age effect less observable (although such an effect with age was seen for CAs). The coefficient for cigarette smoking was 0.0323, indicating that cigarette smokers (on the average) have an 0.0323 increase in SCEs per chromosome. The coefficient for marijuana use is 0.0139, indicating the smaller effect of marijuana use in comparison to cigarettes.

The residuals for the full model (four variables discussed above) are distributed normally, as would be hoped. An interaction term between EDB exposure and marijuana use would test whether an EDB effect on exposure is occurring only in those with marijuana use, and would take the form of a term in the model that was the product of EDB and marijuana use. This term is not significant in the model.

A simple model with just cigarette use (0/1) and marijuana use (0/1) results in an R-square for the model of 0.38, which means that these two variables explain approximately 38% of the variance of the SCE data. An interaction term between cigarette use and marijuana use falls short of significance (p = .17). The coefficient for this term is negative, indicating that the combined effect of smoking marijuana and cigarettes is less than the sum of their individual effects. Hence, the effect modification seen in Table 10.4 (only non–cigarette smokers show a marijuana effect) is evident, but not significant statistically.

The analysis using continuous variables for number of cigarettes smoked and for the frequency of marijuana use show that both of these variables are significant predictors of SCE level. This means that there is a positive dose-response for these variables, strengthening the previously observed associations between SCEs and the dichotomous smoking variables.

Part IV

Surveillance and Screening Studies

Surveillance may be defined as the systematic collection and dissemination of data on disease occurrence. It may also include the collection of data on exposures (hazard surveillance). When the association between exposure and disease is well known, surveillance studies may be particularly appropriate, especially when they can lead to intervention. The intervention will be directed to decreasing the exposure and hence eliminating the disease. For example, surveillance may be appropriate for pesticide poisoning so as to identify where and when it is occurring, leading to possible intervention to eliminate overexposure to pesticides. Another example would be silicosis.

Surveillance studies may also target biologic markers that can be interpreted as either indicators of overexposure or early signs of disease. For example, surveillance of blood leads among lead-exposed workers can detect instances of overexposure and lead to intervention that reduces that exposure.

Medical screening is often conducted primarily to detect early disease for the purpose of providing treatment to the individual (mammography and Pap smear tests are examples of community medical screening). For screening to be useful, practical tests with sufficient sensitivity and specificity must be available, and early detection must be able to lead to effective treatment (for a good discussion, see Hennekens and Buring, 1987). Medical screening in high-risk groups may be thought of as a variant of surveillance if the results of the screening are analyzed for the entire screened group with the intention of public health intervention where needed (Halperin and Frazier, 1985). For example, workers exposed to a suspected bladder carcinogen might be screened for early detection of bladder cancer. If early bladder cancer were detected (in excess), intervention (reduction or elimination of exposure) might be warranted. This kind of study (of a suspected agent) may also be considered an etiologic study, in that the exposure-disease relationship is suspected but not confirmed.

There are three chapters in Part IV. The first is a surveillance study of lead-exposed workers in California, which led to an intervention. The second concerns a screeing study of workers exposed to a suspected bladder carcinogen.

The third is a surveillance study of dermatitis from pesticides in California, which also led to an intervention.

References

Halperin W, Frazier T: Surveillance in the workplace. Ann Rev Public Health 6:419–432, 1985.

Hennekens C, Buring J: *Epidemiology in Medicine.* Boston: Little, Brown, 1987.

Chapter 11 | Occupational Lead Surveillance

ANA OSORIO

Lead intoxication is one of the oldest known occupational diseases. At lower concentrations of lead exposure, there can be nonspecific early symptoms that mimic many other types of illness. These early symptoms include personality changes, fatigue, sleep disturbances, headache, constipation, abdominal pains, and anorexia. At higher lead levels, the later symptoms reflect further involvement of various organ systems:

1. *Hematologic:* anemia, pallor

2. *Gastrointestinal:* severe abdominal cramping ("lead colic")

3. *Neurologic:* peripheral nervous system involvement can result in the inability to extend the hand ("wrist drop"); central nervous system involvement can range from severe headaches to convulsions to coma

4. *Renal:* kidney insufficiency with urinary protein loss and impaired renal clearance

5. *Reproductive:* abortion, developmental abnormalities following in utero exposure, and abnormal semen quality (decreased sperm count, decreased percentage of normally shaped sperm, and decreased number of motile sperm)

There is much individual variability with respect to lead exposure effects. As an approximate guide, the following table lists the blood lead levels (BLLs) at which various medical conditions can occur:

BLL (µg/dl)	Possible Clinical Abnormality
15	Fetal exposure leading to developmental abnormalities in the child
20–35	Increased zinc protoporphyrin (ZPP)*
40	Semen quality abnormalities
40–50	Behavioral changes
50	Low hemoglobin
60–70	More-pronounced behavioral changes
80	Brain damage (encephalopathy)

*ZPP becomes elevated when the synthesis of hemoglobin is blocked by lead. The excess ZPP indicates a biological effect from lead exposure during the prior three months.

Because of the storage of lead in the skeletal system, the BLL in a lead-exposed individual may decrease upon cessation of the exposure, but the skeletal stores will last for years. The primary treatment for occupational lead intoxication is to remove the individual from further lead exposure. For severely symptomatic individuals, chelating agents can be administered to decrease the total body burden of lead.

There is a high risk of lead exposure in: (1) lead battery production, especially for those workers who stack the grids coated with lead paste and those who solder the lead posts and generate lead fumes, (2) radiator repair work, (3) construction or demolition work, especially for those workers cutting lead-painted outdoor structures with acetylene torches (e.g., bridge demolition), (4) reclamation of metal products containing lead (e.g., smelters), and (5) ceramic work using leaded glaze.

A surveillance system is the continual monitoring of either exposure or disease in a given area through the systematic collection and evaluation of relevant data. The goal of an occupational surveillance program is usually intervention to control excessive exposures that can lead to disease. Routine surveillance programs for either exposure or disease are useful when the exposure-disease relationship is well known.

QUESTION 1. Is the testing for BLL an example of the surveillance of exposure or disease? Likewise, how would you classify the ZPP test?

Materials and Methods

Federal Monitoring and Screening Requirements. The Occupational Safety and Health Administration (OSHA) has created a law that sets standards for the biological monitoring and medical screening of lead-exposed workers in the United States.

Once air measurements have established that the air concentration of lead has exceeded or is likely to exceed a specified level (0.03 mg/m^3) for 30 days or more annually, the employer is required to begin medical surveillance. (NOTE: The construction industry is exempt from OSHA lead medical surveillance requirements.) Included in medical surveillance is the testing of the workers for BLL. The frequency of BLL and ZPP testing depends on the initial BLL of the worker. If the initial BLL is less than 40 μg/dl, the BLL and ZPP are obtained every six months. If the BLL is 40 μg/dl or greater, the BLL and ZPP are obtained every two months.

The lead standard states that the individual must be removed from any lead exposure at work (medical removal program) if any of the following situations exist: (1) any BLL is 60 μg/dl or more, (2) a person's average BLL is 50 μg/dl or more for the last three readings, or for all readings during the prior six months (whichever is longer), and (3) the individual has an existing high-risk medical condition such as preexisting renal disease or anemia. The worker may return to his or her job after the BLL is less than 40 μg/dl on two subsequent occasions. When a worker is in the medical removal program, the BLL and ZPP are obtained every month.

QUESTION 2. Can you think of any situations where the above requirements for BLL monitoring might not protect an individual?

California Lead Surveillance. There is no federal lead surveillance program to collect and analyze national occupational BLL information. In 1986, the California state legislature mandated that all laboratories in the state report elevated BLLs to the state health department. These data were to be stored in a California Occupational Lead Registry. Since April 1987, the health department has received laboratory reports for subjects over 16 years of age with a BLL of greater than 25 μg/dl. The reporting form contains the following information: subject's name, address, telephone, employer, and physician. The overwhelming majority of the reports represented occupational exposures. Most of the industries represented in the Registry fell under OSHA BLL requirements, although there were some data for the construction industry that does not come under OSHA BLL requirements (Maizlich et al., 1991).

For individuals with BLLs of 60 μg/dl or greater, from 1988 to 1990 an attempt was made to contact and interview the subject, interview the company and/or personal physician, and, when indicated, interview the employer. Because of funding problems for registry personnel, the 60 μg/dl trigger level and the associated interviews were maintained only through the end of 1990.

QUESTION 3. What are the factors that make a test of BLL a good basis for a lead surveillance system?

Results

In 1988, there were a total of 5,717 reports of subjects with BLLs greater than 25 μg/dl. Since some individuals had repeated values reported, the total number of workers identified was 1,941 (95% were men). There were 133 companies identified through these reports.

QUESTION 4. Why might this surveillance system miss some workers with high BLLs?

Table 11.1 lists the distribution of industry type as percent of total reports to the Registry in 1988.

QUESTION 5. What data are lacking from Table 11.1 that would be useful?

Table 11.2 lists the BLL results as percent of total reports for 1988.
Four percent of the BLLs were above 60 µg/dl. Review of existing data revealed that outdoor building demolition work explained some of these very high BLLs. Registry physicians conducted follow-up of these workers to ensure that they had appropriate medical management. It was decided to study in depth any future cluster of high BLLs in this industry.

QUESTION 6. This is an example of a laboratory-based occupational lead surveillance system. What other sources of information could be used in a lead surveillance system?

A cluster of high lead BLLs among demolition workers soon came to the attention of Registry officials. Two men at a large outdoor demolition worksite were reported to have BLLs above 60 µg/dl BLL.

TABLE 11.1 Industries Reporting Blood Lead Data in California in 1988

Industry	No. of Workers	% of Total
Lead battery	655	44.2
Secondary smelter	373	25.2
Foundries, brass	65	4.4
Firing range	50	3.3
Brass plumbing products	36	2.4
Brass pipe/valves	34	2.3
Brass/copper rolling mill	30	2.0
Pottery	26	1.8
Radiator repair	25	1.7
Foundries, nonferrous	22	1.5

(All other categories <1.5%.)

TABLE 11.2 Blood Lead Levels in California in 1988

Blood Lead Range	No. of Workers	% of Total
<30 ug/dL	838	38.1
30–39	663	36.2
40–49	285	16.9
50–59	89	4.8
60–69	32	1.9
70–79	15	1.2
80–89	12	0.6
90–99	3	0.2
100–109	1	0.1
>109	3	0.1

QUESTION 7. What logical steps should have been taken next by Registry officials?

A physician and an industrial hygienist from the Lead Registry visited the demolition worksite for further information. Twenty-nine men were found to be demolishing a 40 year-old, 380 foot high natural-gas tank that had been repeatedly painted in the past with leaded paint. The two index cases were working as "cutters"; with an acetylene torch, they were cutting the tank into small pieces for removal of the structure and for ease in shipment of material to a metal-reclamation company. Of the 29 men employed, 21 (72%) were cutters and 8 (27%) were noncutters. The average ages of the two groups were 47 and 48 years, respectively, with ranges of 32–64 for the cutters and 25–69 for the noncutters.

Samples of the outer layer of paint on this structure revealed 10% lead content. The permissible exposure limit for airborne lead under the OSHA construction standard is 0.2 mg/m³. Personal breathing zone air samples for lead dust at the worksite had shown concentrations of up to 14 times this allowable level. Because of the potential severity of this lead exposure, it was decided to conduct a more detailed field evaluation of this work force.

The employer already had in place a program of medical screening (physical exam, ZPP), biological monitoring (BLL), and collection of industrial hygiene data (personal sampling for air lead). These "baseline" data were collected while the operation was being performed in the usual manner, prior to the arrival of California Lead Registry officials. Work practices at the time included wearing half-mask respirators with organic vapor cartridges worn during cutting.

With the aim of lowering lead levels, the company then implemented the following changes in work practices.

1. Since leaded paint was found only on the outside tank wall, cutting was done only from the inner surface.

TABLE 11.3 Data for Lead Study*

ID	PREBLL	PREZPP	PRETWA	CUT	POSTBLL	POSTZPP	POSTTWA
1	999	19	999	2	12	24	999
2	50	35	999	1	38	81	999
3	999	12	999	1	999	999	999
4	43	10	1.2	1	999	999	999
5	52	51	999	1	38	72	999
6	34	15	0.62	1	25	22	0.32
7	999	21	999	1	999	999	999
8	83	125	999	1	999	999	999
9	999	21	999	2	999	999	999
10	999	18	0.09	2	27	30	999
11	27	18	0.03	2	999	999	999
12	999	16	0.01	2	999	999	999
13	999	999	0.02	2	19	28	999
14	999	999	999	1	999	999	999
15	59	192	1.72	1	37	999	0.16
16	53	106	999	1	46	227	999
17	999	999	1.54	1	43	160	999
18	51	50	1.18	1	46	90	999
19	48	19	2.85	1	32	69	999
20	69	102	1.2	1	45	999	1.24
21	999	18	999	1	999	999	999
22	24	20	0.67	1	19	23	999
23	999	22	999	1	18	43	999
24	5	4	0.01	2	5	13	999
25	999	18	2.12	1	22	18	999
26	999	999	0.1	1	14	20	0.66
27	999	999	999	1	999	25	999
28	21	8	999	1	999	999	999
29	999	15	999	2	11	13	999

Definitions of variables: PREBLL = pre-intervention BLL (μg/dl); PREZPP = pre-intervention ZPP (μg/dl); PRETWA = pre-intervention time-weighted average for air lead, estimated for an eight-hour work-day; CUT = subject is either a cutter (1.0) or a noncutter (2.0); POSTBLL = post-intervention BLL; POSTZPP = post-intervention ZPP; POSTTWA = post-intervention TWA; 999 = indicates value not available.

*Course instructors may obtain these data on diskette from the editor.

2. Workers started using powered air-purifying respirators.

3. Portable showers and handwashing stands were installed at the work-site.

4. Work coveralls were left at worksite and not worn home.

5. Weekly safety training meetings were begun.

QUESTION 8. What further study might be feasible or indicated at this point?

QUESTION 9. "Post-intervention" breathing zone air lead samples were taken one month after the initial safety and work changes ("intervention") took place. Using the data in Table 11.3, calculate the mean air lead levels for the pre- and post-intervention period, and fill in the table below. (NOTE: the raw data have been somewhat altered for the purposes of this exercise; course instructors may obtain these data on diskette from the editor.) What can you conclude from these results?

Job Category:	Cutter	Noncutter
Number of subjects		
Pre-intervention mean air lead (mg/M³)		
Number of subjects		
Post-intervention mean air lead (mg/M³)		

Construction air lead standard:	0.20 mg/M³*
General industry air lead standard:	0.05 mg/M³*

*For a time-weighted average exposure over an eight-hour work day.

For a better estimate of lead body burden, BLLs were compared pre- and post-intervention. The BLLs of those workers with paired samples were analyzed.

QUESTION 10. Fill in the following table for BLLs before and after intervention for the nine cutters who had data for both times. Comment on the advantages of such "paired" data (for which a paired t-test is used). Comment on the significance of these results.

No. of Pairs	Mean Paired Difference	Std. Err. Mean Difference	t-Statistic, Degrees of Freedom	p-Value

QUESTION 11. Finally, it is important to look at the biological effect that lead may have had on these workers. Fill in the following table for the ZPP levels before and after intervention for the cutters and explain any difference between the BLL and ZPP results.

No. of Pairs	Mean Paired Difference	Std. Err. Mean Difference	t-Statistic, Degrees of Freedom	p-Value

Conclusion

The California Occupational Lead Registry was useful in identifying this lead intoxication outbreak. The follow-up of the index lead intoxication cases led to a field investigation with subsequent industrial hygiene and safety control measures. The ultimate goal of an occupational surveillance program—i.e., intervention to reduce exposures and prevent disease—is well illustrated by this field investigation.

References

Maizlich N, Rudolph L, Royce S, et al.: Elevated blood lead in California adults, 1987–1990. Pub No CDHS (COHP) SR90-001, California Occupational Health Program, California Department of Health Services, Berkeley, 1991.

Waller K, Osorio AM, Jones J: Lead exposure in a tank demolition crew. Submitted for publication, 1992.

Waller K, Osorio AM, Maizlich N, et al.: Lead exposure in the construction industry: results from the California Occupational Lead Registry. Submitted for publication, 1992.

ANSWERS

ANSWER 1. BLL is a reflection of exposure using biological monitoring, and its surveillance is an example of exposure surveillance. An elevated ZPP represents the biological effect from lead exposure, and surveillance of ZPP technically would be considered an example of (early) disease surveillance, based on medical screening data collected in the workplace.

ANSWER 2. (1) Based on the earlier table listing the clinical abnormalities associated with BLLs, there appear to be biological changes that occur below the 50 μg/dl BLL used to institute the medical removal program. Biological monitoring for BLL should not be the primary mode of controlling lead exposure in the workplace. The employer should attempt to prevent lead exposure through engineering controls or replacement of lead-containing products or processes with other ones. A surveillance system can only help alleviate workplace problems that should not have occurred in the first place.

(2) There are worksites where there has been no testing of the air lead levels. In these situations, there is no opportunity for an elevated air lead concentration to trigger the BLL testing. Some occupational medicine specialists feel that a baseline BLL and ZPP should be performed on all workers exposed to lead, whether or not the air concentrations of lead are elevated.

ANSWER 3. BLL is a good test on which to base a lead surveillance system because it is a test that

1. is simple to administer;
2. is relatively inexpensive;
3. does not need highly technical personnel for administration;
4. has a well-established normal range;
5. is a low risk procedure;
6. involves minimal discomfort;
7. is highly reliable and sensitive;
8. is generally required by OSHA for workers with substantial lead exposure;
9. reflects actual body burden rather than potential exposure reflected by air levels;
10. reflects exposure that usually precedes disease, so that when high levels are detected, prompt intervention to reduce levels can prevent disease.

ANSWER 4. If no BLLs are being collected in the workplace, then these workers will never enter the registry. In fact, it is likely that many employers who should be collecting air lead data, and possibly blood lead data, are not doing so (Waller et al., 1991). Furthermore, blood leads might not be collected because air monitoring is inadequate and is not performed during times of peak exposure, or because air monitoring is done but employers are not then complying with OSHA BLL requirements even when blood testing is indicated. If BLL analyses are performed in an out-of-state lab, then these data will be missed by the surveillance program. Another practical problem is that reports are not always filled out completely, and adequate information for follow-up may be missing.

ANSWER 5. There are no estimates of the number of workers at risk by industry (denominators), so that it is impossible to calculate reporting rates and determine whether these rates differ by industry. Different reporting rates might indicate differential compliance with OSHA requirements, or different air lead levels by industry. One industry that is underrepresented in Table 11.1 (less than 1.5% of the total number of reports) is construction, which does not fall under OSHA BLL requirements and in which testing for BLL is less common.

ANSWER 6. Other sources of data might include:

Employer records
Health insurance claims

Workers' compensation claims

National or regional health surveys

Union records

Clinic or hospital records

ANSWER 7. (1) Establish medical status of the two index cases, and ensure worker removal from any lead exposure and appropriate medical treatment.
   (2) Obtain information about other workers who may be similarly exposed/symptomatic.
   (3) Obtain information about work practices and any other hazards.

ANSWER 8. With the consent of the management and the union, a prospective study of the workers was planned, to compare data for BLLs, ZPPs, and air lead measurements before and after changes in work practices. Registry officials administered standardized questionnaires, reviewed medical records, and oversaw the monitoring of subsequent BLLs, ZPPs, and air lead concentrations.

ANSWER 9.

Job Category

	Cutter	*Noncutter**
Number of subjects	10	5
Pre-intervention mean air lead (mg/M³)	1.32	0.03
Number of subjects	4	
Post-intervention mean air lead (mg/M³)	0.60	

*No air lead concentration change were available for the noncutters after intervention.

1. Cutters had a much higher mean air lead level than noncutters.

2. Cutters were exposed to air lead levels, prior to intervention, exceeding the permissible limit. One might argue that air lead levels are not dangerous, assuming appropriate respirator protection is worn at all times during exposure. However, it is preferable to reduce exposures initially rather than rely on respirators. Indeed, BLL data (see Answer 10) indicated that any respirator protection before intervention had been ineffective.

3. Among the cutters, there was a 0.72 unit drop in the mean air lead

concentration following the industrial-hygiene intervention. This indicates that changed work practices (e.g., cutting from the inside, not volatilizing the lead) have effectively reduced the potential for exposure.

4. Even after the intervention, the mean air lead level for the cutters was still above the permissible levels of both the construction (0.20 mg/m³) and the general industry lead standard (0.05 mg/m³).

ANSWER 10.

No. of Pairs	Mean Paired Difference (post-pre)	Std. Err. Mean Difference	t-Statistic, Degrees of Freedom	p-Value (two-sided)
9	−12.66	2.33	5.43, 8 df	.0006

For these nine men for whom there were data before and after intervention, the average pre-intervention level was 44.5 µg/dl blood. Two men had levels greater than 60, while five others had levels above 50. This indicates that whatever respiratory protection was being used, such protection was inadequate, and the high air levels were reflected in high blood levels. After intervention the average for these eight men was 33.1, a significant decrease in BLL. When data are available on the same men before and after some exposure, a paired t-test is appropriate. Paired data are particularly useful for biological outcomes where variability of each individual's physiology (e.g., uptake of lead into the bone, excretion rate via urine) is controlled via the pairing.

ANSWER 11. An *increase* in the mean ZPP is observed after intervention. This increase reflects changes in exposure that occurred up to three months prior to the testing—since ZPP takes longer to rise or fall with exposure than do blood leads. ZPP will be expected to decrease as have the blood leads, with future testing.

No. of Pairs	Mean Paired Difference (post-pre)	Std. Err. Mean Difference	t-Statistic, Degrees of Freedom	p-Value (two-sided)
9	34.33	12.47	2.75, 8 df	.02

References for Answers

Waller K, Osorio AM, Maizlich N, et al.: Lead exposure in the construction industry: results from the California Occupational Lead Registry. Submitted for publication, 1992.

Chapter 12

Bladder Cancer among Chemical Workers

ELIZABETH WARD

In 1981, the National Institute for Occupational Safety and Health (NIOSH) was asked by the Michigan Department of Public Health to investigate the health effects of exposure to 4,4'-methylenebis (2-chloroaniline) (MBOCA) exposure among workers at a small chemical plant in southern Michigan. This plant had come to the attention of State Health Department officials in 1979, when extensive environmental contamination with MBOCA had been discovered in the surrounding community. MBOCA is an aromatic amine with about the same potency as benzidine that is highly carcinogenic in rats and induces bladder tumors in dogs. MBOCA was one of the first fourteen carcinogens for which OSHA promulgated standards in 1974, but the MBOCA standard was withdrawn from consideration for procedural reasons and has never been reinstated (Ward et al., 1987). No adequate epidemiologic studies of MBOCA had been conducted.

NIOSH investigators visited the plan in 1981 to collect information about the history of the process and also obtained records of exposure evaluations in the plant conducted by the Michigan Department of Public Health. In order to evaluate the feasibility of a study of bladder cancer incidence or mortality, investigators copied and computerized personnel records from the plant.

QUESTION 1. How would you use the information collected to determine the feasibility of a study of bladder cancer among workers exposed to MBOCA at this plant?

NIOSH investigators learned that the company had produced MBOCA from 1968 through 1979, initially on a pilot scale. Surveys of urinary MBOCA levels after the MBOCA production process had been shut down in 1979 suggested that MBOCA exposures had been substantial. Moreover, surfaces throughout the plant, including the plant cafeteria, were found to be contaminated with

MBOCA. Since the primary route of exposure to MBOCA is dermal, the surface contamination suggested that all workers in the plant, not just those assigned to the MBOCA process, were potentially exposed.

There were 552 workers identified from the personnel records; most of these were young white males. Almost all personnel records contained adequate information for follow-up, but the information on job assignments was inadequate to differentiate workers by level of exposure. The potential latency period (time since first exposure) averaged 11.5 years, whereas the latency period for most occupational bladder carcinogens averages 20 years. There was also high turnover at the plant, with the median duration of employment being only 3.2 months.

Investigators estimated the number of incident cases and deaths from bladder cancer that would be expected in the population. As of 1983, the year the calculations were done, there were fewer than 0.1 expected deaths from bladder cancer and 0.18 incident cases. The study had 80% statistical power to detect a 35-fold excess risk of bladder cancer mortality and a 16-fold excess risk of bladder cancer incidence.

QUESTION 2. Would you recommend doing a study at this plant? If so, how would you design the study to maximize its public health and scientific value?

Materials and Methods

NIOSH investigators decided to conduct a bladder cancer incidence study. Since there were no long-term cancer registries available in the area where the plant was located, bladder cancer incidence would have to be determined by interview and confirmed by requesting medical records. A practical problem in planning the study was that more than 80% of the study population no longer worked at the plant and 40% no longer resided in the local area. Thus, investigators planned to interview workers by telephone.

A bladder cancer incidence study, unfortunately, was unlikely to discover many bladder cancers in a cohort with this little potential latency. NIOSH also considered initiating a screening program.

QUESTION 3. What are the issues in deciding whether to undertake a screening program for early detection of an occupational disease?

Before deciding to conduct a bladder cancer screening program at this plant, investigators reviewed the literature to determine what screening tests were available and their sensitivity, specificity, and predictive value. There are two screening tests that may be used to screen for bladder cancer (urine cytology and urinalysis or microscopy to detect hematuria). Unfortunately, the literature did not readily yield information on the sensitivity, specificity, and predictive value of these tests. The sensitivity of urine cytology clearly depends on the histologic grade of the tumor. Urine cytology is likely to pick up the higher-grade, more lethal tumors, and less likely to pick up low-grade papillary tumors that have a relatively good prognosis (Farrow, 1990). Examination of the urine for microhematuria may detect some low-grade papillary tumors missed by urine cytology (Messing and Vaillancourt, 1990). The diagnostic examination triggered by a positive test frequently includes both an intravenous pyelogram and a cystoscopy, each of which involve some risk to the patient.

There is no clear evidence from well-designed studies that early detection of bladder cancer reduces morbidity and mortality. However, there is some evidence that, at least for higher-grade tumors arising in workers exposed to aromatic amines, the clinical diagnosis may be preceded by several years of abnormal cytology examinations (Koss et al., 1965).

QUESTION 4. How would you design a study to determine if early detection leads to decreased mortality?

QUESTION 5. Under the circumstances, would you recommend a screening program?

Results

It was decided to conduct both urinalysis and urine cytology, using a testing kit that was mailed to participants' homes. All lab findings would be reviewed by a NIOSH physician, and individuals with suspicious or positive findings would be notified and advised to see their personal physicians.

The interviews and screening examinations began in 1985. Among the 552 workers identified from company personnel records, 452 participated in the telephone interview and 385 participated in the urine screening examination. There were no bladder tumors reported in the telephone interview.

In June 1986, when the urine screening examinations were almost completed, a 28-year-old study participant notified NIOSH investigators that he had been diagnosed with a bladder tumor. In the screening examination, this person had had negative urine cytology and a negative dipstick test for heme (blood) in the urine. However, the red blood cell count on the urinary cytology slide had been slightly elevated (but below the level used by NIOSH researchers to refer patients for diagnostic evaluation), which prompted his personal physician to perform additional urine analyses and cystoscopy. This patient had worked at the plant for one year in 1978, eight years before diagnosis. He had never smoked or been employed in occupations with exposure to bladder carcinogens other than the study plant.

The diagnosis of this tumor was a cause of concern because of the patient's young age and because he had not been referred for diagnostic evaluation based on the criteria used by NIOSH. NIOSH researchers were concerned that there may have been other false negatives using the established criteria. NIOSH investigators therefore decided to offer cystoscopy to approximately 80 individuals who had similar "borderline" screening results and 80 individuals who appeared, based on their interview responses, to have had the higher potential MBOCA exposures. Sixty-five of the 160 individuals offered these examinations elected to participate.

In April 1987, a second tumor was found, after NIOSH-sponsored cystoscopy. This tumor occurred in a 29-year-old man. His earlier screening results had been normal. He had been offered cystoscopy because he was included in the group of workers judged to have had "high" exposure to MBOCA. The patient, who had never smoked, worked at the MBOCA production plant in 1976, 11 years before diagnosis, in jobs that were thought to involve heavy potential MBOCA exposure. The diagnosis of a tumor in a second man under 30 raised concern and suggested that neither the results of prior screening tests nor the exposure ranking scheme could discriminate with confidence between workers who should be offered cystoscopy and workers who were not at high risk. Therefore, it was decided to offer cystoscopy to all workers regardless of their participation status or results in prior studies.

One hundred thirty-nine workers participated in the second round of the screening. These included 15 workers originally selected in the high-risk group and 124 others.

In April 1988, a third worker with a low-grade papillary tumor was diagnosed by cystoscopy. This person was a 44-year-old man whose prior cytology and urinalysis results were negative. He worked in MBOCA production for 1.5 months in 1972, in direct, daily contact with MBOCA. He was a former cigarette smoker who held other jobs in the chemical industry following employment at the MBOCA plant (for a fuller discussion of the results of this study, see Ward et al., 1990).

QUESTION 6. What information would you need to be able to draw conclusions about the carcinogenicity of MBOCA from this study?

Discussion

Although the study results were not definitive, when they were combined with the strong animal evidence of carcinogenicity and MBOCA's structural similarity with other human bladder carcinogens, they increased concern about the ability of MBOCA to cause bladder tumors in humans.

QUESTION 7. What should be done to monitor this population in the future? Should bladder screening examinations be offered again?

References

Farrow G: Urine cytology in the detection of bladder cancer: a critical approach. J Occup Med 32,9:817–821, 1990.

Koss L, Melamud M, Ricci A et al.: Carcinogenesis in the human urinary bladder—observations after exposure to para-aminodiphenyl. N Engl J Med 272:766–770, 1965.

Messing E, Vaillancourt A: Hematuria screening for bladder cancer. J Occup Med 32,9:838–845, 1990.

Ward E, Smith A, Halperin W: 4,4'-Methylenebis(2-Chloroaniline): an unregulated carcinogen. Am J Indust Med 12:537–549, 1987.

Ward E, Halperin W, Thun M, et al.: Screening workers exposed to 4,4'-methylenebis(2-chloroaniline) for bladder cancer by cystoscopy. J Occup Med 32,9:865–868, 1990.

ANSWER 1. There are a number of general questions that should be considered: (1) Is there evidence that the workers were substantially exposed and is there a way to separate the workers by degree of exposure? (2) How long ago did the exposure start and has there been an adequate potential latency to detect an effect if one is present? (3) Was the work force sufficiently stable that there are long-term workers with substantial cumulative exposure to study? (4) How many total workers are potentially involved in the study? Are there complete records to identify all of them? (5) Do the records contain sufficient identifying information to conduct vital status follow-up and/or to contact the workers? (6) Do the records contain sufficient information to determine the duration of exposure for each worker and the departments where they worked? (7) What is the age, race, and sex of the work force? (8) How many cases or deaths from the disease in question would be expected in the population if there were no occupational risk?

ANSWER 2. MBOCA posed a problem frequently encountered in occupational epidemiology. It was a chemical with strong animal evidence for carcinogenicity, had no definitive epidemiologic data, and was not regulated as a carcinogen in the United States. Estimates of the number of workers exposed to MBOCA in the United States range from 1,400 to 33,000 (Ward et al., 1987). As part of the evaluation of whether to do a study at this plant, NIOSH investigators gathered data on other firms producing or using MBOCA in the United States to see if there were better study cohorts. The study plant was one of two U.S. MBOCA producers; the other plan had manufactured known bladder carcinogens such as benzidine. Most of the downstream plants that used MBOCA to manufacture specialty polyurethane products had very small numbers of workers potentially exposed. Thus, while the study plant had many limitations as an epidemiologic cohort, it was determined that it was probably the best one available.

Several ways were considered to maximize the value of the study. These were to study cancer incidence rather than mortality, to design the

study as a prospective one in which workers would be followed periodically in the future, and possibly to conduct bladder cancer screening.

ANSWER 3. The first question to answer in considering a screening
program is to identify and evaluate the screening tests: what tests are
available and what are their characteristics, including sensitivity (the
probability of testing positive if the disease is truly present), specificity
(the probability of testing negative if the disease is truly absent), and
positive predictive value (probability that a person actually has the
disease given that he or she tests positive). Both sensitivity and specificity may be influenced by changing the definition of a positive test,
depending on the investigator's perception of the risks of missing a true
case, benefits of detecting a true case, and risk involved in the procedures for evaluating an individual who tests positive (for a discussion of
these issues, see Hennekens and Buring, 1987).
  In evaluating screening programs, an important issue is whether the
early detection of disease is of benefit to the patient—i.e., is there an
effective treatment available such that early detection results in decreased morbidity or mortality from the disease? A benefit of screening in
the occupational health setting is the earlier recognition of a disease
excess related to an exposure, which may lead to reducing or eliminating
the exposure (Halperin, 1990).

ANSWER 4. Ideally, in investigating the value of a screening program the
best study design would be a randomized trial in which half the participants were assigned to be screened and the other half not to receive
screening (Hulka, 1990). The screened group would be offered bladder
cancer screening examinations periodically. Both groups would be followed for bladder cancer incidence and for deaths from any cause for a
long period (5–10 years minimally). This would be a very difficult and
expensive study. Participants would have to be screened multiple times
and followed over the course of their lifetimes. It is unlikely that a study of
the impact of bladder cancer screening on morbidity and mortality could
be carried out in a high-risk occupational group, first because the group
is likely to be too small and second because it might be unethical to
withhold screening from half of the exposed individuals. However, well-
designed studies in high-risk occupational groups could be useful in
comparing the efficacy of different screening procedures in detecting
bladder cancers.

ANSWER 5. The issues of screening for occupational bladder cancer are
so complex and controversial that they were the subject of a NIOSH-
sponsored symposium in 1989 (Schulte et al., 1990). The reader is

referred to the proceedings of the conference for fuller discussion (J Occup Med 32,9, 1990). The decision to embark on bladder cancer screening in this cohort was based largely on the assumption that screening would enable NIOSH researchers to detect an excess of bladder cancer as early in the latency period for the cohort as possible, and on the hope that screening would be of some individual benefit (i.e., early detection would lead to decreased mortality).

ANSWER 6. To draw a definitive conclusion from this study, you would need information about the prevalence of tumors diagnosed by cystoscopy in asymptomatic persons. This information is not available because cystoscopies are rarely done in asymptomatic persons. Bladder tumors in young men are highly unusual; the incidence of clinically apparent bladder tumors in U.S. males aged 25 to 29 is only 1 per 100,000 per year (Horm et al., 1985).

ANSWER 7. It would be desirable from a public health perspective to continue to monitor cancer incidence and mortality in this population. Mortality follow-up can be accomplished through the National Death Index; cancer incidence data for residents who remain in the state of Michigan may be obtained by record linkage with the Michigan Cancer Registry, which was established in 1985. Although the evidence for the ability of bladder cancer screening to reduce morbidity and mortality from the disease is not available, it would be desirable to offer periodic screening to this cohort. Bladder cancer screening programs are offered to workers exposed to carcinogenic aromatic amines by several large companies. However, in the case of the Michigan plant, very few of the exposed cohort remains employed and the group has dispersed through-out the country. This makes it difficult to conduct a high-quality screening program which provides adequate social support and medical follow-up for individuals with positive tests. One potential benefit of the NIOSH study is that cohort members have been informed of their exposure to MBOCA and their possibly increased risk of bladder cancer. They have been alerted to the symptoms of bladder cancer and advised to see a physician without delay should any of the symptoms occur.

References for Answers

Halperin W (moderator): Where do we go from here? (panel discussion), J Occup Med 32,9:936–945, 1990.

Hennekens C, and Buring J: *Epidemiology in Medicine*; Little, Brown, Boston; 1987.

Horm J, Asire A, Young K, et al. (eds): SEER Program, Cancer incidence and mortality in the U.S. 1973–1981, NIH Publication 85-1837, Washington, D.C., 1985.

Hulka B: Principles of bladder cancer screening in an intervention trial, J Occup Med 32,9:812–816, 1990.

Koss L, Melamud M, and Ricci A et al.: Carcinogenesis in the human urinary bladder—observations after exposure to para-aminodiphenyl, N Engl J Med 272:766–770, 1965.

Messing E, and Vaillancourt A: Hematuria screening for bladder cancer, J Occup Med 32,9:838–845, 1990.

Schulte P, Halperin W, Ward E, et al. (eds): Bladder cancer screening in high-risk groups, J Occup Med 32,9:787–945, 1990.

Ward E, Smith A, and Halperin W, 4,4′-Methylenebis(2-Chloroaniline): an unregulated carcinogen, Am J Ind Med 12:537–549, 1987.

Chapter 13

Occupational
Skin Disease
and Contact
Dermatitis

MICHAEL O'MALLEY

A large number of chemical and physical agents cause either skin irritation or allergy. The constant interaction of skin with the external environment accounts for the fact that occupational skin disease (OSD) represents 40 to 50% of all occupational illness (Nethercott et al., 1986). Classic high-risk industries include landscape and horticultural services; forestry services; poultry processing; leather tanning and finishing; soap, detergent, and cosmetic manufacturing; adhesive manufacturing; and metal plating and finishing (Wang, 1979). The variety of work settings affected illustrates the widespread distribution of potential hazards to the skin.

Contact dermatitis (CD), characterized by redness, blistering, and pruritus (itching) of the skin, accounts for more than 90% of OSD. As the name contact dermatitis implies, the lesions occur in a pattern that matches the contact with either a chemical or physical irritant, or with a skin allergen. Skin allergy represents perhaps 10 to 20% of CD, but accounts for a disproportionate share of cases with long-term disability (Adams, 1990). Skin allergy most often develops after repeated exposure to relatively high doses of an allergenic substance. Once it has developed, an acute response (clinically identical to that produced by irritant contact dermatitis) may occur 24 to 48 hours following exposure to even small doses of the allergen. Accurate diagnosis of allergic CD depends upon a time-consuming and infrequently performed procedure known as the patch test.

Materials and Methods

Use of National and State Surveillance Data for Occupational Skin Disease. Investigators used the Bureau of Labor Statistics (BLS) Annual Survey and data from workmen's compensation agencies to identify cases of occupational skin disease.

The BLS Annual Survey uses the OSHA mandated employers' illness and injury (Form 200) logs to calculate the numerators for incidence rates of OSD and other occupational disorders for a random sample of each Standard Industrial Classification (SIC) in the U.S. work force. Cases recorded include any illness or injury requiring medical treatment beyond first aid. Denominators for the rates are the estimated number of individuals employed in each SIC category (Bureau of Labor Statistics, 1990).

As a companion to the Annual Survey, the BLS maintains a file of workers' compensation reports (based on either reporting by employers or by physicians to designated state compensation agencies), known as the Supplementary Data System (SDS). The criteria for reporting cases of OSD to workers' compensation agencies are based upon either medical treatment for a presumed work-related condition or time lost from work. The specific requirement for reporting lost-work-time cases ranges from one to eight days. SDS data can be broken down by state, and investigators here used SDS data to examine OSD in California.

As might be expected, there is evidence that both the OSHA 200 logs and workers' compensation data greatly underestimate the actual number of cases of OSD (Disher et al., 1975), and there has been considerable debate about the accuracy of these data (Hilaski and Wang, 1982; Wegman, 1985; Whorton, 1983). Despite possible underestimation, these data sources can still be used to determine which industries (by SIC code) have the highest risk of OSD.

Identifying Pesticides that Cause Skin Disease in California.   Data from the Pesticide Illness Surveillance Program (PISP) in California were used to identify particular pesticides causing OSD in that state. Cases identified via the PISP are derived from two sources: (1) pesticide illness reports (PIRs), which are reports by physicians directly to county public health authorities, and (2) Workers' Compensation System cases abstracted from the California Department of Industrial Relations files. Of 3,144 PISP cases reported in California in 1988, 70% were identified only from workers' compensation records, 10% only from PIRs, 13% from both, and 6% by other mechanisms, most often by direct reporting to the County Agricultural Commissioners. These cases included all pesticide illnesses, only some of which was skin disease.

The reported cases of contact dermatitis from PISP surveillance reports were then identified. These were then classified as either definite (contact with known dermatitis-causing agent conforming with pattern of dermatitis), probable (same as above but agent only suspected of causing dermatitis), possible (contact pattern possible, no nonoccupational cause apparent), unlikely (no contact pattern), or unrelated (nonoccupational dermatitis).

Results

National and State Surveillance Data.   Table 13.1 gives rates of OSD from the BLS 1981 Annual Survey (OSHA 200 log) and rates based upon cases reported

TABLE 13.1 1981 Rates of Dermatitis in the Major Industries Measured by the Annual Survey* and the Supplementary Data System

	BLS Annual Survey	SDS Group A (0 LWDs)†	SDS Group B (1–7 LWD)	SDS Group C (8 + LWDS)
Agriculture/forestry/fishing	35.9	43.2	16.3	1.4
Manufacturing	14.8	39.8	3.9	1.9
Construction	8.8	14.1	4.8	1.9
Services	5.8	8.9	2.3	0.6
Transportation	6.5	6.4	2.7	0.4
Mining	4.1	4.3	0.1	0.7
Wholesale/retail trade	2.6	5.8	1.4	0.4
Finance/insurance/real estate	1.3	1.8	0.7	0.2

*Unpublished Annual Survey data obtained from U.S. Bureau of Labor Statistics Bureau of Periodic Surveys; rates are cases/10,000.

†LWD, lost work days required for reporting cases to the SDS. Rates listed are in units of cases/10,000 employed.

From: O'Malley et al., 1988.

to state workers' compensation agencies included in the 1981 SDS file. These data show similar OSD incidence rates for the Annual Survey and compensation claims based upon seeking medical treatment (0 lost work days—Group A). Markedly lower rates are seen for the states reporting only lost-work-time cases (Groups B and C). Despite the quantitative variations in the rates, the relative rankings of industries within each reporting group are similar. Agriculture/forestry/fishing is the industry with the highest rate of skin disease, followed by manufacturing, construction, and services.

To investigate OSD (contact dermatitis) within California agriculture, the data shown in Table 13.2 were assembled, using the SDS file for California agricultural workers (lost-work-time cases). California workers account for a third of total U.S. agricultural employment. Table 13.2 divides the dermatitis data by three broad areas or sources of the dermatitis (plants, agricultural chemicals, food commodities). These categories are unfortunately too broad to provide many clues as to specific etiologies of OSD. For example, the code for "plants" covers both wild vegetation (e.g., poison oak) and crop foliage vegetation. "Chemicals" covers all pesticides and fertilizers, and includes pesticide residues on crops. "Food products" covers all agricultural commodities.

QUESTION 1. In Table 13.2, what is the highest-risk industrial group for dermatitis associated with agricultural chemicals? Plants? Food products?

QUESTION 2. What is the most common source (plants, chemicals, or food products) leading to OSD in California? Does this table help to identify areas with apparent excesses of OSD?

TABLE 13.2 Distribution of Occupational Skin Disease in California Agriculture that Resulted in Lost Work Days by SIC Group* and Source of Exposure

SIC Group	Employed†	Agricultural Chemicals		Plants		Food Products (commodities)		Total	
		Cases	Rate‡	Cases	Rate‡	Cases	Rate‡	Cases	Rate‡
011 Cash grains	26,538	2	0.8	8	3.0	0	0.0	12	4.5
013 Non-grain cash crop	135,401	22	1.6	22	1.6	2	0.1	58	4.3
016 Vegetables/melons	258,492	72	2.8	96	3.7	122	4.7	366	14.1
017 Fruits/trees/nuts	603,615	138	2.3	354	5.9	76	1.3	652	10.8
018 Horticulture	125,826	64	5.1	200	15.9	6	0.5	324	25.7
019 General crop farms	290,856	74	2.5	98	3.4	28	1.0	248	8.5
021 Non-dairy livestock	34,877	4	1.1	14	4.0	2	0.6	24	6.9
024 Dairy farms	61,669	8	1.3	6	1.0	0	0.0	36	5.8
025 Poultry/eggs	41,670	16	3.8	6	1.4	6	1.4	48	11.5
027 Animal specialties	10,571	0	0.0	8	7.6	0	0.0	12	11.3
029 General livestock	10,375	0	0.0	10	9.6	0	0.0	10	9.6
071 Soil prep services	8,046	2	2.5	8	9.9	0	0.0	12	14.9
072 Crop services	177,246	84	4.7	34	1.9	34	1.9	186	10.5
074 Veterinary services	48,931	0	0.0	0	0.0	0	0.0	4	0.8
075 Non-vet animal services	24,309	2	0.8	2	0.8	0	0.0	6	2.5
076 Farm labor services	354,669	60	1.7	144	4.1	52	1.5	304	8.6
078 Landscaping services	127,655	8	0.6	394	30.9	0	0.0	404	31.6
085 Forestry services	2,026	0	0.0	12	59.2	0	0.0	12	59.2
091 Commercial fishing	11,862	0	0.0	0	0.0	0	0.0	0	0.0
Total	2,354,664	556	2.4	1,416	6.0	748	3.2	2,720	11.6

*Based on cases reported to the U.S. Supplementary Data System (for 1978–1981, 1983); restricted to SIC groups with at least 1,000 employees over a five-year period.

†Employment figures from unemployment insurance records by the California Employment Development Department. Reported figures are the sum of mid-third-quarter employment (peak agricultural employment) for the study period.

‡Incidence rates are reported as number of new cases/10,000 workers employed over five years.

From O'Malley et al., 1988b.

Table 13.3 lists pesticides commonly associated with definite, probable, or possible contact dermatitis in California as reported to the PISP system from 1978 to 1983 (the same period covered in Table 13.2). The PISP system for those years did not include SIC codes as part of the case record, so that it was not possible to calculate rates of pesticide-induced skin disease by industry as was done in Table 13.2. The PISP data in Table 13.3 indicate that two chemicals, propargite and sulfur, accounted for 33.8% of the total cases of contact dermatitis.

Further investigation into a specific dermatitis outbreak involving agricultural workers using these two pesticides might indicate the need for a change in work practices. For workers applying pesticides, this most often involves use of protective equipment or closed application systems. But for fieldworkers exposed to residue of pesticides on crop foliage, the principal preventive strategy involves administrative control—requiring workers to stay out of treated fields until the residue has dissipated to a safe level. Implementation of this "reentry interval" strategy demands knowledge of chemical dissipation rates as well as safe residue levels for individual crops and work activities.

Field Investigation of Sentinel Cases.   Via the PISP surveillance system, in June of 1988 the California Department of Food and Agriculture (CDFA) received a report regarding an outbreak of dermatitis among nectarine harvesters (SIC 017) in Tulare County, California (O'Malley, 1990). These harvesters worked with nectarines over a two-week period (June 13–27), and were exposed to propargite as well as other pesticides. Since initial information obtained from the County Agricultural Commissioner's Office indicated no violation of existing reentry intervals had occurred, CDFA investigators sought to determine the cause of the incident. This involved evaluation of numerous sources of potential sources of skin disease known to be present in the agricultural work environment (Adams, 1990; Hogan and Lane, 1986)—including heat, exposure to irritating or allergenic plant materials, and agricultural chemicals.

Among physical agents, the investigation focused on the possible role of excessive environmental heat, since this has previously been postulated to play a major role in the development of dermatitis in California agricultural workers (Winter and Kurtz, 1985).

Dermatitis due to plant allergens was considered to be a less likely cause of the outbreak, since harvesting nectarines does not present an opportunity for contact with poison oak or other noxious weeds and the dermatitis due to nectarines or nectarine foliage has not previously been reported (Mitchell and Rook, 1979).

Several chemical agents had been used on the orchards associated with the outbreak. Propargite was the agent most suspect of causing the outbreak.

The investigation involved administering a brief questionnaire, a review of available medical and work history records, pesticide application data, environmental sampling for pesticide residue, and a brief physical examination.

Forty-six (81%) of the fifty-seven workers in three crews labeled by number as 79, 80, and 89 reported experiencing a rash during the two weeks prior to the interview. No cases were reported among members of a comparison crew

TABLE 13.3 Pesticides Associated with Skin Diseases in California Agriculture: PISP Data 1978–1983*

Pesticide	Cases	Percent of Total
Propargite	241	18.7
Sulfur	195	15.1
Glyphosate	53	4.1
Propargite/sulfur	51	4.0
Methyl bromide	43	3.3
Benomyl	30	2.3
Captan	26	2.0
Petroleum products	24	1.9
Cyhexatin	21	1.6
Captan/sulfur	18	1.4
Dinitrophenol	18	1.4
Ethylene dibromide	15	1.2
Paraquat	15	1.2
Methomyl	13	1.0
Diazinon	12	0.9
Ziram	12	0.9
Captafol	11	0.9
DD mixture	11	0.9
Chlorothalonil	10	0.8
Dicofol	10	0.8
Captan/DCNA/Sulfur	9	0.7
Acephate	8	0.6
Carbaryl	8	0.6
DCNA	8	0.6
Malathion	8	0.6
Naled	8	0.6
Dienochlor	8	0.6
Triadimefon	8	0.6
Dimethoate	6	0.5
Fenbutatin oxide	6	0.5
Anilazine	5	0.4
Benomyl/captan	5	0.4
Maneb	5	0.4
Simazine	5	0.4
Metam-sodium	5	0.4
Zineb	5	0.4
Other	168	13.0
Unknown	184	14.3
Total	1,288	100.0

*Pesticide Illness Surveillance Program, operated by the California Department of Food and Agriculture. 1982 omitted.

working in the same area, labeled as number 86. Thirty-three (72%) of those reporting a rash sought medical treatment, and medical records were obtained for thirty-two (97%) of these workers. The reported dates of onset ranged from June 18 to June 27, although no workers sought medical treatment until June 23. Twenty-five workers (75.7% of those seeking treatment) reported visiting a physician on June 25. Interview with the employer revealed that this large group was sent for evaluation after a case of blistering facial dermatitis was recognized in one of the members of crew 89.

Of the 46 workers who reported a rash on the questionnaire, the rash was confirmed to be contact dermatitis in 42 (91%) by physical examination, either at the time of initial treatment or at the time of the CDFA examination. Three cases of contact dermatitis among members of the three affected crews were identified on examination in individuals who had not reported a rash during the interview. The specificity of the questionnaire in identifying a rash confirmed to be contact dermatitis on medical examination was thus 82% (19/23) and the sensitivity was 93% (42/45).

QUESTION 3. Using clinical examination as the standard for comparison, what is the predictive value of a report of dermatitis on the questionnaire?

The suspect orchards where the crews had been working prior to illness were sampled for possible pesticide residues. A small number of dislodgeable residue samples were collected by cutting 5-cm discs out of the leaves. The samples were then assayed for the three chemicals most recently applied to the trees: propargite, formetanate hydrochloride, and iprodione. Measured levels of formetanate hydrochloride ranged from 0.30 to 1.26 $\mu g/cm^2$ at the time of sampling for affected crews. Three samples of iprodione showed no detectable levels and a fourth showed a trace (0.91 ppm). The estimated levels of propargite ranged from 0.55 to 1.91 $\mu g/cm^2$ for affected crews. The unaffected crew worked in propargite-treated orchards for three days; the estimated level of propargite-dislodgeable residue ranged from 0.14 to 0.82 $\mu g/cm^2$. They also worked in ten orchards treated either with formetanate hydrochloride or *B. thuringiensis,* but no residue samples were available from these fields. Between June 13 and June 27 the high daily temperature ranged from 90 degrees (June 21) to 103 degrees (June 19).

Table 13.4 lists the data for the three affected crews and the one unaffected crew, for the two-week period in which they were working in the orchards in question (course instructors may obtain these data on diskette from the editor). Days of exposure to propargite, formetanate hydrochloride, *Bacillus thuringiensis,* and iprodione are shown for each individual, as well as the days working in untreated fields prior to the onset of rash. For subjects who did not report a rash, exposures reflect exposure over the entire two-week period. Using the data from the leaves regarding residues of propargite, by orchard, an estimated cumulative exposure (residue/days) to propargite was also calculated for each individual (PresHrs). Workers could be exposed to more than one pesticide per day. Some workers worked less than 14 days.

TABLE 13.4 Case Listing of Day of Rash Onset and Important Exposure Variables*

Crew	PresHrs	Pdays	Fdays	Undays	Idays	Bdays	Degdays	Rash
80	15.78	2	2	3	0	0	83	1
80	15.78	2	2	3	0	0	83	1
80	15.78	2	2	3	0	0	83	1
80	21.29	3	3	3	0	0	94	1
80	50.74	6	5	3	1	0	135	1
80	15.78	2	2	3	0	0	83	1
80	32.60	5	5	3	1	0	117	1
80	57.30	7	5	3	1	1	147	0
80	50.74	6	5	3	1	0	135	1
80	32.60	5	5	3	1	0	117	1
80	26.52	4	4	3	0	0	104	1
80	32.60	5	5	3	1	0	117	1
80	21.29	3	3	3	0	0	94	1
80	15.78	2	2	3	0	0	83	1
80	50.74	6	5	3	1	0	135	1
80	57.30	7	5	3	1	1	147	0
80	15.78	2	2	3	0	0	83	1
89	25.55	5	5	1	1	0	101	1
89	60.52	9	8	1	2	0	153	1
89	31.07	6	6	1	1	0	112	1
89	31.07	6	6	1	1	0	112	1
89	67.07	10	8	1	2	1	169	0
89	67.07	10	8	1	2	1	160	1
89	31.07	6	6	1	1	0	112	1
89	36.29	7	7	1	1	0	122	1
89	60.52	9	8	1	2	0	153	1
89	60.52	9	8	1	2	0	153	1
89	60.52	9	8	1	2	0	153	1
89	25.55	5	5	1	1	0	101	1
89	27.11	6	6	1	1	0	112	1
89	60.52	9	8	1	2	0	153	1
89	60.52	9	8	1	2	0	153	1
89	42.37	8	8	1	2	0	135	1
89	60.52	9	8	1	2	0	153	1
89	31.07	6	6	1	1	0	112	1
89	36.29	7	7	1	1	0	122	1
79	16.82	3	3	6	1	0	135	1
79	16.82	3	3	6	1	0	135	1
79	5.51	1	1	6	0	0	112	1
79	16.82	3	3	6	1	0	122	1
79	34.96	4	3	6	1	0	153	0
79	34.96	4	3	6	1	0	153	0
79	34.96	4	3	6	1	0	153	0
79	5.51	1	1	6	0	0	112	1
79	34.96	4	3	6	1	0	153	0
79	16.82	3	3	6	1	0	122	1
79	34.96	4	3	6	1	0	153	0
79	34.96	4	3	6	1	0	153	1
79	34.96	4	3	6	1	0	153	1
79	16.82	3	3	6	1	0	122	1
79	34.96	4	3	6	1	0	153	1

(continued)

TABLE 13.4 Case Listing of Day of Rash Onset and Important Exposure Variables*
(*Continued*)

Crew	PresHrs	Pdays	Fdays	Undays	Idays	Bdays	Degdays	Rash
79	34.96	4	3	6	1	0	153	0
79	34.96	4	3	6	1	0	153	1
79	34.96	4	3	6	1	0	153	0
79	10.74	2	2	6	0	0	122	1
79	34.96	4	3	6	1	0	153	0
79	34.96	4	3	6	1	0	153	1
86	6.11	3	8	4	0	2	169	0
86	6.11	3	8	4	0	2	169	0
86	6.11	3	8	4	0	2	169	0
86	6.11	3	8	4	0	2	169	0
86	6.11	3	8	4	0	2	169	0
86	6.11	3	8	4	0	2	169	0
86	6.11	3	8	4	0	2	169	0
86	6.11	3	8	4	0	2	169	0
86	6.11	3	8	4	0	2	169	0
86	6.11	3	8	4	0	2	169	0
86	6.11	3	8	4	0	2	169	0
86	6.11	3	8	4	0	2	169	0
86	6.11	3	8	4	0	2	169	0
86	6.11	3	8	4	0	2	169	0
86	6.11	3	8	4	0	2	169	0
86	6.11	3	8	4	0	2	169	0
86	6.11	3	8	4	0	2	169	0
86	6.11	3	8	4	0	2	169	0
86	6.11	3	8	4	0	2	169	0

*Crenum = crew number; Preshrs = hours of exposure * estimated propargite residue; Pdays = days in propargite-treated fields; Fdays = days in formentenate hydrochloride-treated fields; Undays = days in untreated fields; Idays = days in iprodione treated fields; Bdays = days in fields treated with *Bacillus thuringiensis*; Degdays = (daily maximum temperature −80) × number of days worked; Rash = 1 for yes, 0 for no.

Note: All workers worked from June 13 to June 17. All time variables truncated at time of rash occurrence. Course instructors may obtain these data on diskette from the editor.

QUESTION 4. Calculate the mean cumulative exposure to propargite (PresHrs), as well as the mean Pdays, Idays, Fdays, Bdays, and Undays among the three affected crews versus the one unaffected crew (#86), and comment on the results. Among the three affected crews, does the probability of rash increase with increasing average cumulative exposure to propargite (PresHrs)? Among the affected crews, determine the mean PresHrs for those with a rash and those without a rash. Comment on the results.

QUESTION 5. The above analysis indicates that the three affected crews had higher duration of exposures to propargite and iprodione (Pdays and

Idays). Calculate the correlation coefficient between Pdays and Idays for all workers. Is it possible to statistically separate the two exposures? Based upon the residue information, which compound appears to be the most likely cause of the outbreak? Is this consistent with previous information about the causes of dermatitis in California agricultural workers?

Discussion

The apparent cause of the high incidence of dermatitis in the three crews was determined to be residues of propargite that persisted well beyond the two-day orchard reentry interval. Subsequent to the outbreak described above, propargite was identified as a possible female reproductive hazard, based upon finding of maternal toxicity on oral administration to pregnant rabbits. Together with concerns about dermatitis, this prompted extension of the existing post-application field reentry period from 2 to 21 days on stone fruit and to 30 days on grapes, effective as of the 1989 harvest. The data in Table 13.5 (based on PISP data) indicate the apparently successful effect of this intervention on reported cases of dermatitis.

TABLE 13.5 Possible, Probable, and Definite Contact Dermatitis Associated with Field Residue Exposure to Propargite as the Primary Pesticide— Grapes and Tree Fruit 1982–1990*

Year of Illness	Crop	
	Grapes	Tree Fruit†
1982	12	0
1983	18	1
1984	38	0
1985	21	1
1986	0	133
1987	3	3
1988	4	60
1989	1	0
1990	0	1

*Source: Pesticide Illness Surveillance Program (PISP)— see text for description.

†Tree fruit includes nectarines, peaches, citrus, plums, and prunes. The 1986 cases in tree fruit derive from a single cluster of dermatitis in citrus harvesters exposed to an extended release form of propargite. The 1990 data are partial, based on entry of 2,868 of 2,922 case reports.

QUESTION 6. Based upon the data in Table 13.5, extension of the reentry intervals for propargite appears to have had a dramatic effect on the number of cases associated with exposure to propargite. Given the concerns about underreporting of OSD, can you suggest a means of confirming the apparent low rate of propargite-induced dermatitis?

References

Adams RM: *Occupational Skin Disease,* 2nd edition. Philadelphia: Saunders, 1990.

Bureau of Labor Statistics, U.S. Department of Labor. Employment and Wages Annual Averages, 1989. Bulletin 2373. Washington, D.C., 1990.

Discher D, Kleinman G, Forster F: Pilot study for development of an occupational disease surveillance method, HEW Publ. No (NIOSH) 75-162, Washington, D.C., 1975.

Hilaski HJ, Wang CL: How valid are estimates of occupational illness? Monthly Labor Review: 27–35, August 1982.

Hogan D, Lane P: Dermatologic disorders in agriculture. State of the Art Reviews in Occupational Medicine 1:285–300, 1986.

Mitchell J, Rook A: *Botanical Dermatology—Plants and Plant Products Injurious to the Skin.* Vancouver: Greengrass, 1979.

Nethercott JR, Gallant C: Disability due to occupational contact dermatitis. State of the Art Reviews in Occupational Medicine 1:199–203, 1986.

O'Malley M, Thun M, Morrison J, Mathias CGT, Halperin WE: Surveillance of occupational skin disease using the supplementary data system. Am J Indust Med 13:291–299, 1988.

O'Malley M, Mathias CGT: Distribution of low-work-time claims for skin disease in California agriculture: 1978–83. Am J Indust Med 14:715–720, 1988b.

O'Malley M, Smith C, Krieger R, Margetich S: Dermatitis among stone fruit harvesters in Tulare County, 1988. Am J Contact Dermatitis 1:100–111, 1990.

Wang CL: Occupational skin disease continues to plague industry. Monthly Labor Review: 17–22, February 1979.

Wegman D: Surveillance needs for occupational health. Am J Pub Health 75:1259–1261, 1985.

Whorton M: Accurate occupational illness and injury data in the US: can this enigmatic problem ever be solved? Am J Pub Health 73:1031–1034, 1983.

Winter CK, Kurtz PH: An investigation into factors influencing grape worker susceptibility to skin rashes. Bull Env Contam Toxicol 35:418–426, 1985.

ANSWERS

ANSWER 1. Horticulture; forestry services; vegetables; melons.

ANSWER 2. Plants are the source of most OSD in California. These data, while not sufficiently precise to be used as a basis for intervention, do provide at least an initial guide to the agricultural sectors in which OSD rates are highest. Some interesting leads can be observed. For example, in hostricultural specialities (SIC 018), the large number of plant-related claims probably is the result of dermatitis subsequent to exposure to cut flowers that are allergens, such as primroses, chrysanthemums, daisies, lilies, and poinsettias.

ANSWER 3. Predictive value is the proportion of true cases among reported cases. A total of 46 cases had positive responses to the questionnaire, and 42 of these had a positive finding of CD on clinical examination (predictive value 91%).

ANSWER 4.

Means	Affected Crews	Unaffected Crews
PresHrs	34.4	6.1
Pdays	5.0	3.0
Fdays	4.5	8.0
Idays	1.0	0.0
Bdays	0.1	2.0
Undays	3.4	4.0

The affected crews had high duration and estimated cumulative exposure to propargite (PresHrs) compared to the unaffected crew, and high duration of exposure to iprodione (the unaffected crew had none). The reverse trend was seen for other variables (including Degdays). The exposures were not independent, so that increasing days in orchards treated with propargite (for example) resulted in fewer days in fields treated with bacillus or formetanate hydrochloride. Note that the exposures of the unaffected crew were all the same—they all had identical work histories over the two-week period.

The above data show that exposures to propargite and/or iprodione were apparently associated with the occurrence of dermatitis.

The mean PresHrs for crews 79, 80, and 89 were 26.7, 31.1, and 46.1, while the probability of rash increased from 62%, to 88%, and to 95% for these three crews. These data are consistent with a dose-response, with increasing cumulative exposure to propargite resulting in increasing incidence of dermatitis. However, the mean PresHrs for the 46 rash cases was actually lower (32.6) than the mean PresHrs for the 11 individuals without rash (41.9). This may reflect individual susceptibility. Those individuals who were not susceptible to getting a rash in the affected crews did not get a rash over the two-week period, while the duration measures for those who did get a rash were truncated at the time the rash occurred. Thus, those few individuals in the most affected crews who did not get a rash have a high number of days of exposure (and hence high cumulative exposure) to propargite.

ANSWER 5. Propargite and iprodione were often used on the same orchards, resulting in a high correlation (r = 0.89). It is not possible to ascertain if either exposure was a separate risk factor while controlling for the other, using multivariate analysis. However, the mean exposure to iprodione was less than one day in the group with the rash and negligible levels of iprodione were found in the field at the time of the field investigation. Propargite is a known skin irritant, as demonstrated by the 1978–83 data in Table 13.5, as well as the results of skin irritation tests in rodents demonstrating the corrosive nature of propargite. Animal tests indicate that iprodione is a moderate skin irritant (O'Malley, 1990). Hence, it appears more likely that propargite, rather than iprodione, was responsible for the outbreak.

ANSWER 6. Periodic examination surveys of workers in fields treated with propargite would provide data on the incidence and prevalence of dermatitis. While no such data exist for earlier years for comparison, it would at least be possible to ascertain the dermatitis rates are now low among workers working in fields previously treated with propargite.

Measures and Statistics

Measures, Tests of Association, and Test-based Confidence Intervals for 2 × 2 Tables, One Stratum

Assume the data are organized in contingency tables as shown (from Kleinbaum, Kupper, and Morgenstern, 1982) in Tables A.1 and A.2 (the index "g" represents a stratum).

Consider Table A.1. When there is only one stratum the subscript "g" can be ignored. In this case, the relative risk (Table A.1) between exposed and nonexposed is $(a/n_1)/(b/n_0)$. Relative risks may be calculated in cohort studies with

TABLE A.1 Count Data (cohort studies with count data, case-control studies, cross-sectional studies)

	Diseased	Not Diseased	
Exposed	a_g	c_g	n_{1g}
Not exposed	b_g	d_g	n_{0g}
	m_{1g}	m_{0g}	n_g

TABLE A.2 Person-Time Data (cohort studies with person-time data)

	Diseased	Person-Time
Exposed	a_g	L_{1g}
Not exposed	b_g	L_{0g}
	m_{1g}	L_g

count data, or in cross-sectional studies. The odds ratio is ad/bc. Odds ratios are calculated in case-control studies and may also be calculated in cross-sectional studies.

The chi-square (one degree of freedom) for testing the association for the data in Table A.1 is often expressed as the sum over all four cells of [(observed-expected)^2/expected]. An equivalent formula somewhat easier to compute is:

$$\chi^2 = n(ad - bc)^2/(a + b)(c + d)(a + c)(b + d)$$

The calculated chi-square can then be compared with a tabulated chi-square distribution with one degree of freedom, to determine the probability (p-value) of having obtained the observed chi-square (or a more extreme value), under the null hypothesis.

Consider Table A.2, and again consider only one stratum, so that the subscript "g" is ignored. The rate ratio for cohort studies with person-time data is $(a/L_1)/(b/L_0)$. The chi-square test of association (one degree of freedom) for the data in Table A.2 is

$$\chi^2 = [a - (m_1 L_1/L)]^2/(m_1 L_1 L_0/L^2)$$

This test assumes a large sample size, such that $m_1 L_1/L$ and $m_1 L_0/L$ (the expected number of cases in exposed and nonexposed under the null hypothesis) are each at least 5.

Chi-square tests of association test the null hypothesis of no difference between exposed and nonexposed. It is often preferable, however, to present instead a range of plausible values for the measure of interest (e.g., the odds ratio). This can be done by calculating confidence intervals for the measure. Test-based confidence intervals are easily calculated by hand from the corresponding chi-square statistics presented above; 95% test-based confidence intervals for relative risks, odds ratios, or rate ratios are:

Lower limit = ratio measure$^{(1 - 1.96/x)}$

Upper limit = ratio measure$^{(1 + 1.96/x)}$

The reader should be aware that test-based intervals are approximate, and are more inadequate as the observed data depart strongly from the null hypothesis (see Kleinbaum et al., 1982 for a discussion of other types of confidence intervals).

Measures, Tests of Association, and Test-based Confidence Intervals for 2 × 2 Tables, More than one Stratum

When there is more than one stratum, as when the data are stratified by level of a potential confounder, Mantel-Haenszel–type relative risks, odds ratios, and rate ratios (Kleinbaum et al., 1982) may be calculated as below:

$$\text{Relative risk} = \sum_{g=1}^{G} \frac{a_g\, n_{0g}}{n_g} \bigg/ \sum_{g=1}^{G} \frac{b_g\, n_{1g}}{n_g}$$

$$\text{Odds ratio} = \sum_{g=1}^{G} \frac{a_g\, d_g}{n_g} \bigg/ \sum_{g=1}^{G} \frac{b_g\, c_g}{n_g}$$

$$\text{Rate ratio} = \sum_{g=1}^{G} \frac{a_g\, L_{0g}}{L_g} \bigg/ \sum_{g=1}^{G} \frac{b_g\, L_{1g}}{L_g}$$

The Mantel Haenszel chi-square (one degree of freedom) test of overall association for relative risks and odds ratios is shown below, without any continuity correction:

$$\chi^2 = \left(\sum_{g=1}^{G} \frac{a_g d_g - b_g c_g}{n_g} \right)^2 \bigg/ \sum_{g=1}^{G} \left(\frac{n_{1g} n_{0g} m_{1g} m_{0g}}{(n_g - 1)(n_g)(n_g)} \right)$$

The Mantel-Haenszel chi-square (one degree of freedom) test of overall association for rate ratios (person-time data) is:

$$\chi^2 = \frac{\left(\sum_{g=1}^{G} a_g - \sum_{g=1}^{G} (m_{1g} L_{1g}/L_g) \right)^2}{\sum_{g=1}^{G} \frac{m_{1g} L_{1g} L_{0g}}{(L_g)(L_g)}}$$

Test-based confidence intervals for the respective measure may be calculated using these chi-square statistics.

Below we present an example of the calculation of these measures and statistics for hypothetical data from a cohort study (count data).

	Young			Old		
	Dis	Not Dis		Dis	Not Dis	
Exp	10	30	40	55	50	105
Not Exp	15	105	120	50	75	125
	25	135	160	105	125	230

The Mantel-Haenszel χ^2 (one degree of freedom) is

$$\frac{\left(\dfrac{(105)(10) - (30)(15)}{160} + \dfrac{(55)(75) - (50)(50)}{230}\right)^2}{\dfrac{(40)(120)(25)(135)}{(159)(160)(160)} + \dfrac{(105(125)(105)(125)}{(229)(230)(230)}} = 6.43 \ (\text{p-value} = .01)$$

The Mantel-Haenszel relative risk is

$$\frac{\dfrac{(10)(120)}{160} + \dfrac{(55)(125)}{230}}{\dfrac{(15)(40)}{160} + \dfrac{(50)(105)}{230}} = \frac{7.50 + 29.89}{3.75 + 22.83} = 1.41$$

The 95% test-based confidence interval for the relative risk is (1.08, 1.83).

Standardized Rate Ratios

An alternative method of controlling for confounding in cohort studies is via either direct or indirect standardization, methods often used in cohort studies with person-time data. In standardization, the rate ratio in each stratum is weighted to derive a summary rate ratio. The formula for the rate ratio is:

$$\frac{\displaystyle\sum_{i=1}^{W} w_i \text{rate}_{1i} \bigg/ \sum_{i=1}^{W} w_i}{\displaystyle\sum_{i=1}^{W} w_i \text{rate}_{2i} \bigg/ \sum_{i=1}^{W} w_i}$$

In this formula, rate_1 is the rate for exposed and rate_2 is the rate for the nonexposed. The index, i, ranges from 1 to W and indexes the strata, which typically will categorize the rates by age, sex, race, and calendar time, as well as other possible confounders. Notice that the weights are the same for both the exposed and nonexposed populations (the rates have been "standardized").

In indirect standardization the weights, w, are the person-years of the exposed population. Indirect standardization is often used in cohort mortality studies. The resulting summary measure, called the SMR, or standardized mortality ratio, is often expressed as the ratio of observed deaths to expected deaths.

In direct standardization the weights are often that of a large external population, such as the U.S. population. Sometimes the weights are taken to be the combined person-year distribution of the exposed and nonexposed population. Directly standardized rate ratios have one advantage over indirectly standardized rate ratios—namely, that several of them can be mutually compared, as long as they have all been calculated using the same set of weights. This is not true of indirectly standardized rate ratios, since for each of them the weights differ.

Consider the following example for standardized rate ratios.

Age	Rate ratio	Nonexposed		Exposed		Weights (indirect)	Weights (direct)
		Deaths	Person-yrs	Deaths	Person-yrs		
<45	1.00	5	500	2	200	200	700
45–64	1.00	6	300	6	300	300	600
>55	2.00	6	200	30	500	500	700
Totals		17	1000	38	1000		

The crude rate ratio is 38/17, or 2.24. The indirectly standardized rate ratio is

$$\frac{\dfrac{(2/200)200 + (6/300)300 + (30/500)500}{1000}}{\dfrac{(5/500)200 + (6/300)300 + (6/200)500}{1000}} = 38/23 = obs/exp = 1.65$$

The directly standardized rate ratio is

$$\frac{\dfrac{(2/200)700 + (6/300)600 + (30/500)700}{2000}}{\dfrac{(5/500)700 + (6/300)600 + (6/200)700}{2000}} = 1.53$$

The Mantel-Haenszel rate ratio for these same data is 1.49. Note that all three summary rate ratios differ (depending on the weights used), and none is inherently more valid than another.

SMRs are often calculated when the nonexposed population is very large in comparison to the exposed population, so that the rate in the nonexposed may be taken as invariant. It is then possible to treat the sum of the observed over all cells as a Poisson variable (Σa_g). Using the notation of Table A.2, the overall expected is the sum of $b_g L_{1g}/L_{0g}$ over all strata, which is taken as the mean of a Poisson distribution. In this situation a chi-square test of significance of the SMR, with one degree of freedom (Armitage, 1973), may be used to test whether the total observed differs significantly from the total expected for SMRs. The test (presented here with a continuity correction) is based on the normal approximation to the Poisson distribution. Under the null hypothesis, the test statistic (shown below) is distributed as a chi-square (one degree of freedom):

$$\chi^2 = \frac{(|observed - expected| - 0.5)^2}{expected}$$

Trend Test for SMRs. Sometimes the investigator is interested in assessing whether the data exhibit a dose-response trend. This is usually done by determining if there is a positive linear trend in disease as exposure level increases. For person-time data, the incidence rate is compared among exposure groups (e.g., nonexposed, low exposure, high exposure). Mutually comparable directly standardized rates are best for comparison across exposure categories. However, indirectly standardized rate ratios (SMRs) may also be compared by a simple chi-square test (one degree of freedom) described by Breslow et al. (1983). Results will usually parallel those obtained using directly standardized rates. The data layout for the test is as below, where the $E_j{}^*$ are the "adjusted" expected deaths calculated so that they maintain the same proportions across the "J" exposure categories as the original expected deaths, but their sum now equals the sum of the observed.

$$\sum_j E_j^* = \sum_j O_j$$

	Exposure Category			
	1	2	...	J
Observed deaths	O_1	O_2	...	O_J
Expected deaths	E_1	E_2	...	E_J
Expected deaths (adjusted)	E_1^*	E_2^*	...	E_J^*
Exposure level (score)	z_1	z_2	...	z_J

$$\chi^2 = \frac{\left(\sum_j z_j(O_j - E_j^*)\right)^2}{\sum_j z_j^2 E_j^* - \left(\sum_j z_j E_j^*\right)^2 \Big/ \sum_j O_j}$$

For example, for the data below, the chi-square testing for a positive trend in SMRs across latency categories is $9139.36/8532.00 - 6517.87) = 4.54$, with a p-value of 0.03.

	Exposure Category		
	1	2	3
Observed deaths	9	14	13
Expected deaths	12.70	14.35	7.39
Adjusted expected deaths	13.28	15.00	7.72
SMR	0.71	0.97	1.76
Average latency (yr)	5	15	25

Trends for Count Data. If the data are count data rather than person-time data (i.e., case-control data, cross-sectional data, or a cumulative incidence cohort study), an increasing trend in disease across exposure categories may be tested via the Mantel-extension test (1983). This is a test for a linear trend in proportions, and is illustrated below, following the presentation by Rothman (1986). The letter j indexes the exposure. The data shown below illustrate only one stratum (i) of a confounding variable(s), but the formula for the test uses the index, i, to denote as many strata as needed. The test may be used for data that are not stratified by ignoring the summation over i.

Exposure Category

	0	1	2	. . .	j
Cases	a_0	a_1	a_2	. . .	a_j
Noncases	b_0	b_1	b_2	. . .	b_j
Total	N_0	N_1	N_2	. . .	N_j

The chi-square test (one degree of freedom) for a linear trend in proportions of diseased subjects across exposure categories is:

$$\chi^2 = \frac{\left[\sum_i \left(\sum_j a_j x_j - \left(\sum_j a_j \Big/ \sum_j N_j \right) \sum_j N_j x_j \right) \right]^2}{\sum_i \left\{ \left[\left(\sum_j a_j \sum_j b_j \right) \Big/ \left(\sum_j N_j \right)^2 \left(\sum_j N_j - 1 \right) \right] \left[\sum_j N_j \sum_j N_j x_j^2 - \left(\sum_j N_j x_j \right)^2 \right] \right\}}.$$

In the above (rather complicated) formula, the x_j represents the score assigned to each exposure level (e.g., 5 ppm, 15 ppm). This formula collapses to the usual Mantel-Haenszel chi-square test for association if there are only two exposure levels. Also, any stratum i with 0 cases or controls is noninformative and should not be included in the calculation.

The use of this formula is illustrated in the data below, to test for a (linear) trend for disease risk with increasing duration of employment.

Exposure Category

	0	1	2	3
Cases	45	48	72	56
Controls	75	52	67	36
Total	120	100	139	92
Average duration of employment (yr)	0	6.0	14.5	20.5

In these data there is an increasing trend in the proportion of diseased with increasing duration of employment. The chi-square statistic (one degree of freedom) is $(274.16)^2/(.000555)(11,977,473) = 11.30$, which has a probability $p < .005$.

Trend Test for Odds Ratios Obtained from Logistic Regression. Analysis of case-control data (and sometimes cumulative incidence cohort data) is often done via logistic regression. Logistic regression is a mathematical model in which the observed outcome is dichotomous (0 if control, 1 if case). The goal of the model is to predict the outcome as a function of predictor variables that may be either categorical or continuous. If exposure is categorized in logistic regression, the model will yield a coefficient β and estimate of the odds ratio (e^β) for each level of exposure, typically versus the lowest exposure category (often no exposure). Often, in such cases, the investigator may wish to assess whether there is a linear increasing trend in such odds ratios as the exposure level increases. Exposure levels must be assigned by the investigator, and may be the midpoint of exposure categories (if exposure is a continuous variable), or a simple ranking (e.g., 1, 2, 3). The slope of such a linear trend may be estimated by the formula below, from Rothman (1986). In this formula the w_j's are the weights (the inverse of the variance of the odds ratios), the x_j's are the exposure scores (often the midpoints of the exposure categories), and the or_j's are the odds ratios for the j categories. The variance of the odds ratio is approximately equal to the square of the odds ratio multiplied by the variance of the coefficient β as derived from logistic regression. In the calculations, the reference category (e.g., the nonexposed) is omitted.

$$\text{slope} = \frac{\sum_j w_j x_j or_j - \sum_j w_j x_j}{\sum_j {}_j x_j^2}$$

and

$$\text{std err(slope)} = \sqrt{\frac{1}{\sum w_j x_j^2}}$$

By way of example, consider the following data.

	Exposure category			
	None	Low	Medium	High
β	—	0.30	0.50	0.70
Odds ratio (or_j)	1.00	1.35	1.65	2.01
Std error β	—	0.25	0.20	0.30
Variance odds ratio	—	0.114	0.109	0.364
Weights (w_j)	—	8.79	9.17	2.75
Exposure level (x_j)	0	1	2	3

In this example the slope is 0.33 and its standard error is 0.12. The 95% confidence interval is (0.09, 0.57), indicating a positive trend in the odds ratio with increasing exposure.

A word of caution is in order regarding all the above tests for linear trend. These tests are not tests for a monotonic dose response, and they can in some instances overstate the case for a positive dose response (see Maclure and Greenland 1992). Inspection of the data for reasonably consistent increases of response with dose must accompany any statistical test.

Analysis of Matched Data

Matching is often done in case-control studies, as a means to control confounding more precisely than otherwise. Matching refers to the practice of choosing cases and controls so that they have the same values for certain factors thought a priori to be confounders. For example, one control might be selected for each case (pair-matching), such that the control was of the same sex, the same age, and had the same smoking habits as the case. Alternatively, several controls can be matched to each case (r-to-1 matching).

The analysis of matched data is done by stratifying on the matching variable(s), which simply means treating each matched set (either a pair, or one case with multiple controls, or all cases and controls in a matched category if frequency matching has been used) as a separate stratum. Then the Mantel-Haenszel measures and tests of association described in Part 1 can be calculated. Often this kind of stratified analysis will involve a large number of strata. For pair-matched data, an equivalent method for calculating the Mantel-Haenszel odds ratio and test statistic is shown below. In the data layout shown below, each case-control *pair* is treated as a single observation. The odds ratio is the ratio of discordant pairs, b/c. The chi-square test statistic is called the McNemar's statistic and is $(b - c)^2/(b + c)$.

		Control		
		E	Not E	
Case	E	a	b	$a + b$
	Not E	c	d	$c + d$
		$a + c$	$b + d$	n

Sample Size Calculations

It is usually important, prior to beginning any study, to estimate the sample size that will be needed to detect a given level of risk, should such a level exist. In case-control studies this means estimating the number of cases and controls needed to detect a given (hypothesized) odds ratio. One generally wishes to have a certain statistical power (usually 80%) to reject the null hypothesis in a study, under the assumption that the true odds ratio to be detected in fact is elevated above the null value of 1.0.

To calculate sample size, the investigator must (1) hypothesize an odds ratio he or she wishes to be able to detect with high probability, (2) estimate the expected prevalence (P_0) of the exposure among the controls (given (1), one can then calculate the estimated prevalence among cases, P_1), (3) determine his or her desired power to detect the hypothesized odds ratio (probability of rejecting the null hypothesis when the alternative hypothesis is true ($1 - \beta$), and (4) determine his or her desired probability of rejecting the null hypothesis if the null hypothesis is true (α). The necessary number of controls (n_0) for an unmatched case-control study may then be computed by the following formula (Rothman and Boice, 1979), for a given ratio (R) of cases to controls (this same formula can used for cumulative incidence cohort studies):

$$n_0 = (Z_\beta^2 K + Z_\alpha^2(A + B)^2 + 2Z_\alpha Z_\beta(A + B)\sqrt{K})/(P_1 - P_0)^2(A + B)$$

Here $A = P_1(1 - P_0) + P_0(1 - P_1)$, $B = (R - 1)P_0(1 - P_0)$, and $K = (A + B)(RA - B) - R(P_1 - P_0)^2$, Z_β is the cumulative standard normal distribution corresponding to the desired power (e.g., $Z_\beta = 0.84$ corresponds to power = 0.80 and $\beta = 0.20$), and Z_α is value of the standard normal distribution corresponding to the desired rejection level (e.g., if $\alpha = .05$, $Z_\alpha = 1.96$). For example, suppose we want to be able to detect an odds ratio of 1.7 with an exposure prevalence of 10% among controls, corresponding to a case exposure prevalence of approximately 16%. Assuming a 1-to-1 ratio of cases to controls (so that $B = 0$), the needed sample size is 486 cases and 486 controls.

Chi-square Test of Association for Tables Larger than 2 × 2

The chi-square test of association presented for the 2 × 2 table can be extended to larger (r rows by c columns) tables. The formula is

$$\chi^2 = \sum \frac{(observed - expected)^2}{expected}$$

The summation is over all r × c cells, and the chi-square statistic has $(r - 1) \times (c - 1)$ degrees of freedom. For example, suppose the investigator wishes to determine whether the exposed and nonexposed have different smoking habits, after observing the data below.

	Never-smokers	Former smokers	Current smokers	
Exposed	20(17.5)	20(20)	40(42.5)	80
Nonexposed	15(17.5)	20(20)	45(42.5)	80
	35	40	85	160

The expected (shown in parenthesis in the table) can be derived for each cell from the marginal totals. The sum of (observed-expected)^2/expected over all six cells equals 1.01, which is a chi-square statistic with 2 degrees of freedom (p = 0.60).

Elementary Statistics for Continuous Outcomes

Some studies involve outcomes that are not "disease" versus "nondisease" but rather are continuous variables such as lung function or nerve conduction velocity. In this situation it is common to compare the mean value of the exposed group to the mean of the nonexposed group via a t-test. The formula for the two-sample t-test is shown below:

$$t_{n_1+n_2-2} = \frac{(\bar{x}_1 - \bar{x}_2) - 0}{\text{std err}(\bar{x}_1 - \bar{x}_2)}$$

The standard error in the above denominator is as follows:

$$\sqrt{\frac{((n_1 - 1)s_1^2 + (n_2 - 1)s_2^2)}{n_1 + n_2 - 2}} \sqrt{\frac{1}{n_1} + \frac{1}{n_2}}$$

where $(n_1 + n_2 - 2)$ are the degrees of freedom of the t-statistic. The s_j's are the sample variances for each group, as shown below for s_1^2:

$$s_1^2 = \frac{\sum_{i=1}^{n_1} (x_{i1} - \bar{x}_1)^2}{n - 1}$$

where the x_{i1}'s are the individual values in the first sample.

By way of example, consider the following data:

Group 1:   65   66   53   68   56   77   72   68   55   67   51   62   77
Group 2:   54   68   74   49   61   58   51   62   63   78   72   58

Here the mean of group 1 is 64.38, the mean of group 2 is 62.33, the difference in sample means is 2.05, s_1^2 is 73.76, $s_2^2 = 83.88$, the standard error of the difference of means = 3.55, the t_{23} statistic is 0.58, and the p-value (for a t this large or larger, two-sided) is 0.57.

The t-test assumes that observations in each group are distributed normally, and that the variances in the two groups are approximately equal. For very small sample sizes, nonparametric tests are preferred.

There is also a t-test for paired samples. In this test the outcome is measured on a number of paired study subjects (e.g., paired to be of the same age, race, and sex). Often the "pair" is a single person tested before and after some exposure. In this test, the differences in the outcome variable for each pair (D) are averaged and the t-test ($n - 1$ degrees of freedom) determines whether the mean difference (D) is different from zero (the null hypothesis is that the differences are 0). The following formulas are needed:

$$\text{var}_D = \frac{\sum_{i=1}^{n} (D_i - \bar{D})^2}{(n - 1)}$$

$$t_{n-1} = \frac{\bar{D}}{\sqrt{\dfrac{\text{var}_D}{n}}}$$

The sample correlation coefficient may be calculated when one wishes to determine the degree to which two continuous variables are correlated (linearly related). The formula for the sample correlation coefficient (Pearson's) is:

$$r = \frac{\sum_{i=1}^{n} (x_i - \bar{x})(y_i - \bar{y})}{\sqrt{\left[\sum_{i=1}^{n} (x_i - \bar{x})^2 \right] \left[\sum_{i=1}^{n} (y_i - \bar{y})^2 \right]}}$$

The correlation coefficient (r) varies from -1 to 1, with 1 indicating perfect positive correlation, 0 indicating no correlation, and -1 indicating perfect negative correlation. Two variables can be related strongly but not in a linear fashion. In these cases the sample correlation coefficient may be near 0; without careful interpretation, this may mislead the investigator to conclude that the two variables are not related.

CHI-SQUARE TABLE

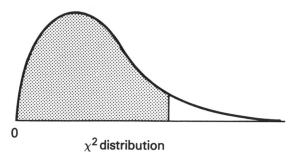

0

χ^2 distribution

Percentiles of the Chi-Square Distribution (shaded area)

% d.f.	0.5	1	2.5	5	10	20	30	40	50
1	0.0001	0.0002	0.001	0.004	0.016	0.064	0.148	0.275	0.455
2	0.010	0.020	0.051	0.103	0.211	0.446	0.713	1.022	1.386
3	0.072	0.115	0.216	0.352	0.584	1.005	1.424	1.869	2.366
4	0.207	0.297	0.484	0.711	1.064	1.649	2.195	2.753	3.357
5	0.412	0.554	0.831	1.145	1.610	2.343	3.000	3.655	4.351

% d.f.	60	70	80	90	95	97.5	99	99.5	99.95
1	0.708	1.074	1.642	2.706	3.841	5.024	6.635	7.879	12.116
2	1.833	2.408	3.219	4.605	5.991	7.378	9.210	10.597	15.202
3	2.946	3.665	4.642	6.251	7.815	9.348	11.345	12.838	17.730
4	4.045	4.878	5.989	7.779	9.488	11.143	13.277	14.860	19.997
5	5.132	6.064	7.289	9.236	11.070	12.833	15.086	16.750	22.105

References

Armitage P: *Statistical Methods in Medical Research.* London: Blackwell Scientific Publications, 1973.

Breslow N, Lubin J, Marek P, et al.: Multiplicative models and cohort analysis. J Am Stat Ass 78,381:1–12, 1983.

Kleinbaum D, Kupper L, Morgenstern H: *Epidemiologic Research.* Belmont, California: Lifetime Learning Publications, 1982.

Maclure M and Greenland S. Tests for trends and dose-response: misinterpretation and alternatives. Am J Epidemiol 135: 96–104, 1992.

Mantel N: Chi-square tests with one degree of freedom: extensions of the Mantel-Haenszel procedure. J Am Stat Assoc 58:690–700, 1963.

Rothman K: *Modern Epidemiology.* Boston: Little, Brown, 1986.

Rothman K, Boice J: *Epidemiologic Analysis with a Programmable Calculator,* NIH Publication 79-1649, U.S. Government Printing Office, Washington, D.C. 20402, 1979.

Index